Holistic
Reflexology

"*Holistic Reflexology* presents in detail a large number of new possibilities to take advantage of the virtues of reflexology. Not to be missed by anyone who already knows and appreciates the value of reflexology or by those who want to discover this wonderful technique!"

CHRISTOPHER VASEY, N.D., AUTHOR OF
THE ACID-ALKALINE DIET FOR OPTIMUM HEALTH

"Ewald Kliegel's work is a wonderful exploration into the world of our microcosms and reflex zones. *Holistic Reflexology* is an invaluable resource for anyone seeking to understand what their body is trying to communicate with an itch, ache, pain, or blemish, and how it may be balanced. I highly recommend this comprehensive text for healing arts practitioners, their clients, or anyone wanting to better know and support the health of their body."

BRIDGETTE SHEA, L.AC., MAcOM,
ACUPUNCTURIST, CHINESE MEDICINE PRACTITIONER,
AYURVEDA EDUCATOR, AND AUTHOR OF
HANDBOOK OF CHINESE MEDICINE AND AYURVEDA

HOLISTIC REFLEXOLOGY

Essential Oils and Crystal Massage in Reflex Zone Therapy

Ewald Kliegel

Healing Arts Press
Rochester, Vermont

Healing Arts Press
One Park Street
Rochester, Vermont 05767
www.HealingArtsPress.com

Healing Arts Press is a division of Inner Traditions International

Note to the reader: This book is intended as an informational guide. The remedies, approaches, and techniques described herein are meant to supplement, and not to be a substitute for, professional medical care or treatment. They should not be used to treat a serious ailment without prior consultation with a qualified health care professional.

Library of Congress Cataloging-in-Publication Data

Names: Kliegel, Ewald, 1957- author.

Title: Holistic reflexology : essential oils and crystal massage in reflex zone therapy / Ewald Kliegel.

Description: Rochester : Healing Arts Press, [2018] | Includes bibliographical references and index.

Identifiers: LCCN 2018002947 (print) | LCCN 2018004237 (ebook) | ISBN 9781620557532 (pbk.) | ISBN 9781620557549 (ebook)

Subjects: LCSH: Reflexology (Therapy) | Essences and essential Oils— Therapeutic use. | Crystals—Therapeutic use.

Classification: LCC RM723.R43 K57 2018 (print) | LCC RM723.R43 (ebook) | DDC 615.8/224—dc23

LC record available at https://lccn.loc.gov/2018002947

Printed and bound in the United States by Versa Press, Inc.

10 9 8 7 6 5 4 3 2 1

Text design by Virginia Scott Bowman and layout by Priscilla Baker
This book was typeset in Garamond Premier Pro with Cocomat, Futura, and Avenir used as display typefaces
Illustrations by Ewald Kliegel, photography by Ines Blersch

To send correspondence to the author of this book, mail a first-class letter to the author c/o Inner Traditions • Bear & Company, One Park Street, Rochester, VT 05767, and we will forward the communication, or contact the author directly at **www.reflex-balance.eu.**

Contents

3

Diagnosis

4
Techniques

5
Holistic Reflexology Treatments

A Holistic Approach

Almost everyone knows reflexology of the feet or at least has heard of it. You may have already received such a massage, or perhaps you take care of others' health and well-being with these kinds of treatments. Reflexology, however, encompasses a much wider range, far beyond just the feet. There are ways we can alleviate headaches with gentle oil rubs into the elbow, regulate diarrhea or constipation with massages on the lower limbs, and improve function following stroke with massage on certain areas on the head, sometimes even years after the initial stroke. All of these are reflexology treatments too; they are just largely unknown, and so until now only a relatively small circle of enthusiastic practitioners has made use of these possibilities. In short, the various reflexology systems outlined in this book are maps of health. They allow us to identify and treat internal disturbances externally. In the twenty reflexology systems found in the body from the head to the feet, the organs can be addressed in a variety of ways to relieve pain, to improve chronic conditions, to communicate with the essence of our organs, or simply to relax.

This book is the result of forty years of experience as a medical masseur, a natural healer, and a lecturer. I would like to share with you my longtime fascination with the many methods of natural healing and invite you to accompany me into the world of reflexology. First let me offer my sincere thanks to the Healing Arts Press team for helping me clearly express myself in the English language. I am so grateful for their hard work and their support of this project.

In this book you will become familiar with a rainbow of possibilities and not least learn more about yourself. The strategies for everyday complaints and the tips on how to use these systems have expanded over the years as more and more people are discovering the efficacy of reflexology. Nevertheless, after all this time I am still touched by the great possibilities our skin holds for us, and sometimes I think I'm the greatest learner of all.

Enjoy with me the miracles of reflexology!

1

......

Introduction to the World of Reflexology

NOTHING NEW UNDER THE SUN

Reflexology is not new. It may in fact be among the most ancient treatment methods of humankind. Ötze, the iceman found in the Tyrolean Alps, is our witness. On his 5,300-year-old mummy are tattoos on his skin that show certain acupuncture points that have been confirmed by experts in acupuncture. This shows that the shamans of our European ancestors who lived at the end of the Stone Age had knowledge about health issues that equaled that of their contemporaries in China and India who were practicing traditional Chinese medicine (TCM) at that time. From this we may assume that all high cultures over the past few thousand years have developed external treatment methods via the skin. This knowledge seems to be a worldwide phenomenon, with unique characteristics in each culture.

For example, according to legend, about six thousand years ago the mystic Chinese emperor Huang Ti brought forth the meridians as an energetic system in which the flow of energy through the body can be regulated by means of certain points on the surface of the skin that are activated by way of special needles or special massages. Ancient ayurvedic doctors found another way. They discovered what amounts to transformer stations in our bodies that supply the right voltage to every organ. We can compare this to a simple kitchen appliance, the electric mixer. Suppose we could connect the mixer to a 10,000-volt power line. When we turn the mixer on the resulting explosion would probably blast our house away. On the other hand, say we are much more careful and connect the mixer to a 1.5-volt battery. Of course nothing would happen, since the power source is too low. Basically the ayurvedic healers had the same principle in mind when they said that humans float in an ocean of energy like fish in water, hence the "transformer stations," the chakras, which regulate

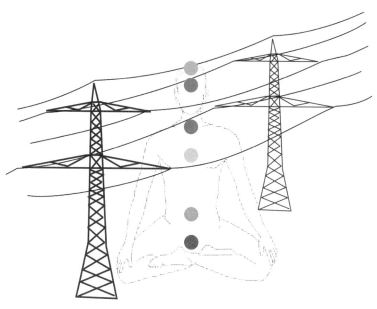

The chakras serve as a kind of transformer station to regulate energy to our organs.

the power supply to our organs so that we have neither too much nor too little.

Unlike the ancient Chinese and Vedic peoples the Celtic culture on the European continent had no written records; therefore knowledge was transmitted as part of an oral tradition. There the main bearers of health knowledge were the druids, a priest- and priestess-hood that appears in legends as wizards and magicians. The demise of the druids came as a result of the strict prohibition of the practice of Celtic (pagan) spirituality by the Roman emperor Tiberius (42 BCE–37 AD) and his successors. Into this power vacuum the Romans could expand their empire without great resistance, and so the last remnants of the ancient knowledge were wiped out within a few short centuries, and the mostly female bearers of that knowledge were burned in the fires of the Inquisition.

Knowledge, however, is never lost; it always comes back in a contemporary form. This is especially true of the timeless achievements of humankind. After the Roman imperial culture, European explorers and conquerors tried to expand their cultural dominance to other areas of the world. For this they needed maps, which in the course of time became more and more accurate, and with these they set about exploring the last remaining unexplored areas, right on up to the twentieth century. In this intellectual environment incredible inventions appeared to further our knowledge. With the advent of technology like microscopes and telescopes the empirical scientific approach got a big boost, allowing us to see more and more of the fine details of material existence.

By the middle of the nineteenth century the first reflexology systems were articulated and described as maps on the skin. At first the reflexology systems of the feet and the hands were used independently as practitioners didn't consider the fact that they related to similar maps found in other parts of the body, such as in the nose or on the back.

It was only from about 1970 on that this more or less dualistic approach evolved into a more holistic way of thinking, in which it was found that various systems could be integrated to address the body, mind, emotions, and spirit.

A MODERN RENAISSANCE:
HOW EVERYTHING BECAME NEW

The first modern systematic descriptions of reflexology zones came from the American brothers W. and D. Griffin, who wrote in 1834 about body disorders and spinal responses. Sixty years later, in 1893, English physician Henry Head described dermatomes, the relationships between the segments of the spinal column and the zones of the skin. That same year Scottish physician Stephen McKenzie discovered sclerotomes, the assignments of the bones to the segments of the spinal column, where the spinal segments have a clear representation on the skin. Both Head and McKenzie were knighted for their contributions.

The first modern writings on hands—including some hints about reflexology of the hands—are attributed to Philipus Meyens, whose book *Chiromantia medica* (medical palmistry) was published in Dresden in 1670. This is considered one of the earliest works on reflexology.

In 1873, Hungarian physician Ignaz von Peczely assigned various signs in the iris to the organs in his treatise *A szivárványhártyáról* (About the Iris). But even earlier than that, in 1724, the Chinese emperor Qianlong (Qing Dynasty) discovered a system in the eyes.

In 1883 the German-Polish physiologist Rudolph Voltolini recognized that certain zones in the nose correspond to the sexual organs. Voltolini concluded from his studies that the functions of the sexual organs could be associated with certain zones in the nose. This assumption turned out to be right, and about ten years later a German professor of gynecology, Wilhelm Fliess, used these zones very successfully in his work at the Charité hospital in Berlin. By etching these zones in the nasal mucous membrane with cocaine base, the complaints and disorders concerning the reproductive organs of his female patients disappeared. By 1950 the German physician Niels Krack was able to achieve this same success by substituting essential oils for cocaine. Unfortunately this application has become largely consigned to history, but today a form of therapeutic "nose drilling," in which the inside of the nose is gently massaged with cotton swabs, is still practiced.

In the early 1900s came the advent of foot reflexology as elucidated by American doctor William Fitzgerald, who in 1917 wrote of his experiences in the book *Zone Therapy*. He observed the foot massages practiced by Native Americans and compared their treatments with his Western knowledge of anatomy. In doing so he perceived a system on the feet and described it in fine detail. In 1924, American physician Joe Shelby Riley complemented Fitzgerald's findings with his book *Zone Reflex*. Fitzgerald and Riley's innovation was not massage of the feet—after all, other earlier cultures such as the Egyptian,

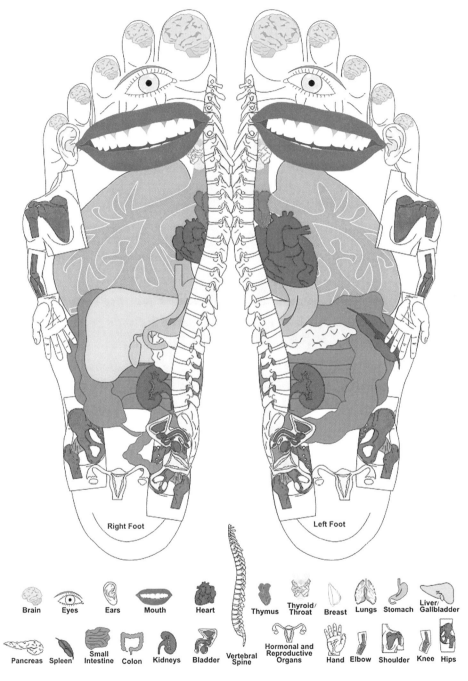

A reflexology map on the soles of the feet

the Chinese, the Maya, the Vedic, the Persian, and the Celtic, also massaged the feet. The new thing was the recognition of a clear system that can be transferred to every human, in which it is possible to identify the organs precisely via a coordinate system. The practical implementation of this system took place a short time later with the work of American physiotherapist Eunice Ingham, who developed a system of massage strokes that spread all over the world in the following decades.

Another landmark in reflexology came some thirty years after the discovery of dermatomes, when German physiotherapist Elizabeth Dicke brought theory to practice in a very personal way. One of her legs was scheduled to be amputated because of blood-flow disorders. With the date of the surgery already set, she started to massage the skin of her lower back with plowlike strokes. She felt a tingling sensation in the lower leg that became especially intense the deeper she plowed her fingers. Her lower limb began to revitalize through this method of massage, and she was able to avoid the need to amputate the limb. This massage technique, which she perfected over the years, became the connective-tissue massage. This massage is performed in the dermatomes and targets the reflexology connections between the skin and the attributed spinal segment. It can be used to improve breathing and digestion, relieve tensions, or, as in Dicke's case, regulate blood circulation. Nowadays connective-tissue massage is a regular part of the curriculum of massage therapists and physiotherapists everywhere. In fact this technique was my introduction to reflexology in 1976, an interest and enthusiasm that has never waned.

Scientific interest in reflexology accelerated in the latter part of the past century. In 1950, French neurologist Paul Nogier discovered a map of the organs in the ears. Nogier's discovery led to increasing interest in and research on the efficacy of auriculotherapy, or ear reflexology. During the 1960s the Japanese scientist Toshikatsu Yamamoto found two reflexology systems on the scalp. In the 1970s Austrian physician Hans Zeitler discovered a reflexology system on the skull, while Chinese biologist Zhang Yingqing discovered a new biological discipline called ECIWO, "embryo-containing information of the whole organism," a bioholographic law that allowed for the identification of hundreds of new acupuncture and reflexology points. In the 1980s Russian researcher Alexander Kachan documented a system of reflexology zones in the area of the nose and the lips via electrical measurements. And German natural therapist Rudolf Siener described reflexology zones on the lower limbs in 1988. Around this same time Korean doctor Tae Woo Yoo published his book *KHT Koryo Hand Therapy* on hand reflexology, and in 2003 another Korean physician, Park Jae Woo, published *A Guide to Su Jok Therapy,* yet another approach to hand reflexology.

There have been many other essential discoveries made in the past fifty years. In the 1970s the German brothers Voll and Peter Mandel made an important contribution to the fundamental understanding of reflexology with their approach to electro-accupuncture, the measuring and stimulation of certain acupuncture points with electrical impulses. In 1983, German physician and dentist Joachim Gleditsch was one of the first to publish a holistic view of reflexology that showed parallels to traditional Chinese medicine. In 2007, French doctor Martine Faure-Alderson applied the concept of embryonal germ layers—groups of cells in an embryo that contribute to the formation of all organs and tissues—to her reflexology work. A complete holistic approach for physical, emotional, and mental health, this includes the whole human energetic system with correspondences to acupuncture, naturopathy, the chakra system, homeopathy, and even the role of the cerebrospinal fluid in craniosacral therapy. And American reflexology pioneers Kevin and Barbara Kunz, who have authored a number of books on the subject, have conducted extensive research on foot reflexology, developing a huge database of scientific studies that are included as part of their seminars, treatments, and books. All of these scientists, practitioners, doctors, and natural healers have contributed valuable new discoveries to the field of reflexology that have broadened its applications for both chronic conditions and for general well-being. So what began as an arcane discipline 150 years ago is now an accepted holistic treatment modality.

THE HOLISTIC NATURE OF REFLEXOLOGY

One of the most fascinating aspects of the human body is the fact that there are so many of these reflexology maps found on different parts of the body. By reading the zones that are located on the surface of the skin on different parts of the body we can discover incipient health disturbances, which may otherwise remain hidden, before they become chronic problems. Most of the time these are not severe problems, unless we ignore the signs.

For example, a pimple on the face on the right side of the nose, an itching on the right shoulder, or a red spot on the lower right side of the rib cage on the front of the torso—these are all signs that the liver and gallbladder are stressed. If we ignore these signs and continue

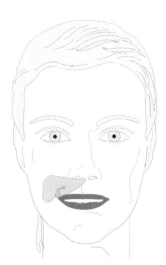

Reflexology of the liver and gallbladder on the face

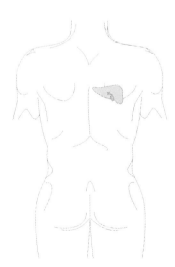

Reflexology of the liver and gallbladder on the back

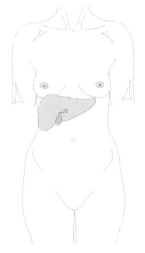

Reflexology of the liver and gallbladder on the front

an inappropriate lifestyle consisting of fatty meat and booze, too much anger, and not enough rest, the signs of distress will become more blatant. Eventually the pimple will disappear, but the pain on the back of the shoulder blade will increase to the point that the gallbladder will need emergency medical intervention.

Reflexology presents us with an open book on one's state of health that is waiting to be read, thus awakening us to our full human potential for self-healing. Reading the reflexology maps found at different locations on the body means understanding what's going on at a deeper level. To make optimum use of this great self-healing resource, intuition comes into play as we read the maps. This doesn't mean that common sense is disregarded—we need our analytic abilities to sort out our perceptions and findings to give our treatments useful direction. It's the combination of both the heart and the brain that opens us to new dimensions of treatment. But intuition plays a far greater role in healing than one might imagine.

Let's consider some new brain research by German physicist Gunther Haffelder. He proved that the analytical side of the brain, located in the left hemisphere, has a processing speed of about 20,000 bits per second in a sequential mode, while the right hemisphere, which is responsible for our feelings and intuitions, processes data at a speed of 60,000,000,000 bits per second in parallel with the left hemi-

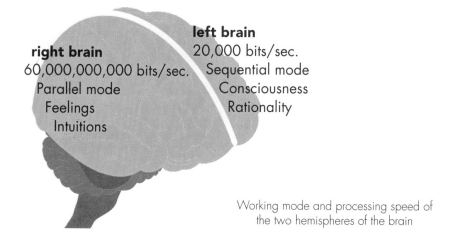

right brain
60,000,000,000 bits/sec.
Parallel mode
Feelings
Intuitions

left brain
20,000 bits/sec.
Sequential mode
Consciousness
Rationality

Working mode and processing speed of
the two hemispheres of the brain

sphere. This proves that intuition has a formidable role in cognition, far beyond the esoteric or aesthetic. Whether one's orientation tends more toward the rational or more toward the intuitive, reflexology has advantages for both types of people. Rationalists may understandably reject the spiritual aspects of the zones on the hands, but they are fascinated by the neurological elegance of the dermatomes and sclerotomes. Many intuitive people feel that the scientific explanations of the zones on the back or on the ears do not conflict with the concept of holism and the fact that we possess microcosms within the macrocosm that is the body. With reflexology, rationalists discover a whole world that is not rationally explainable, while intuitives learn that the practice of reflexology requires a rational component.

Reflexology proves that we are holistic creatures, and every attempt to separate parts from other parts causes problems. The head is connected to the toes, and it gives them orders via the nerves as to what movement to perform. The pancreas produces the hormone insulin, which reaches from the tip of the nose to the end of the little toes. The holistic principle extends even further. In addition to the holism of the body there is a coherence between the mind and the soul. When we are excited we feel it all over. Even the hair gets a better shine. On the other hand, depression is clearly visible in one's posture and face. If you're depressed you can do whatever you want to improve your hair, but it will still remain dull. There are many more examples of the holism of the human being. Those who live their lives with a sense of purpose seem to sparkle out of every cell, and they are obviously satisfied with life. It is equally obvious when someone is unhappy and living without a sense of purpose. And so the expressions of a person are evidence that every part of a human being is interdependent with every other part. Any disturbance within will have an effect on the whole body, and this is where the skin comes into play, as it provides us with a system whereby we can assess the condition of our inner organs. Reflexology allows us to observe on the outside what happens on the inside. Now that red spot on the shoulder blade has a meaning that we can interpret as a dysfunction of the gallbladder. Our intuition might have already told us this long before we were consciously aware of it, but now we can back up our intuition by reading the maps and using our rational sense to recognize the problem.

A MAP OF ABUNDANCE FROM THE HEAD TO THE TOES

Maps are not the actual territory they describe, but they do orient us to an area. Above all, maps are most useful when they help us find our way. As a map of human health reflexology shows us the location of the organs on our skin and how to get in contact with them. If we possessed only one of these systems it would be a stroke of luck, but we are equipped with many of these maps of health, microcosms of the macrocosm, and every one of them has its own specialty. To express it differently: With a satellite fertility map of a geographic area we are able to decide whether to grow apples or grain there. But to drive from New York to L.A., only a road map will bring us there efficiently, while a completely different kind of map is needed to undertake a mountain hike in the Rockies. We can understand the maps of reflexology in the same way. To recognize various emotional-physiological types we need a face map. A back map shows us whether organs suffer from stress, a front map allows us to see how one copes with emotional problems, and an ear map gives information about where our body's power supply and energetic impulse situation is experiencing problems.

Reflexology offers insights that can help us diagnose a problem and also offers great treatment solutions. When we use the reflexology maps at our disposal we can better help clients stay healthy, and we also gain a valuable method for maintaining our own health and well-being. With reflexology we are able to hear what the organs are trying to tell us as well as how to react to this information; hence reflexology enhances our inner communication. Reflexology is nearly always able to improve someone's condition in situations of crisis, and it is a great system for enhancing health and well-being. It awakens our inner healer, which is capable of transforming the imbalances of disease conditions into the balanced condition of health. Anyone can use reflexology. Professional physiotherapists and chiropractors can use it to estimate the precision of the sclerotomes. Podiatrists already have the feet and lower legs in their hands as part of their practice, so reflexology provides them with additional knowledge. In other professions people perform reflexology massage sometimes without even realizing it. By massaging the skull, forehead, and occiput of their clients, hairdressers provide supporting impulses to the whole body. The effects are well known: relaxation and a deep sense of well-being. Other kinds of energetic healers have a wealth of possibilities at their disposal when they incorporate reflexology, as reflexology zones are special gateways into our energetic sphere.

Last but certainly not least, reflexology offers a great choice for self-treatment of everyday ailments. Reflexology can be used by anyone, on anyone, with only one caveat: treatments should never be painful. Discomfort is a sign to reduce the intensity of the treatment.

READING THE SIGNS

When we begin our study of reflexology and its zone systems our experiences sometimes seem to be contradictory. For example, let's assume we get an active reflexology zone concerning the gallbladder on the front of the torso, but there is no such observable sign on the back. The explanation would be that this person tends to react with anger, since the front side indicates the emotional aspects of the organs. The physical organ itself may be unaffected by this tendency; therefore the back system is silent. But if this emotional state is prolonged eventually the person will suffer from problems with the gallbladder. At that point the back will sound its alarm to show on the outside what is happening on the inside. With this example we can see that every reflexology system has a different range of application, as shown in the following table.

REFLEXOLOGY SYSTEMS AND THEIR PROPERTIES

Reflexology System	Main Structures	Influences
Skull	Mainly face, hands, arms, and feet	Muscular activity sensitivity, nervous impulses, blood circulation, musculoskeletal system, follow-up area for stroke
Occiput and forehead	Musculoskeletal system and sensory organs	Pain relief, chains of muscle controls, follow-up area for stroke
Neck	Cervical spine, autonomous nervous system	Pain relief, problems resulting from dislocation of cervical spine
Lymphatic neck points	Lymphatic flow in the neck	Lymph congestion in sinus, tonsils, ears, teeth, throat
Lymph belt	General lymphatic flow	Lymph congestion
Iris of the eyes	Mirror of the whole person in body and soul	Shows physical and emotional dispositions
Face	Inner organs	Deficiencies and dispositions
Ears	Whole body, neurological software	Nerve connections and inner communication
Nose bridge	Musculoskeletal system and selected organs	Vertebral spine, pain relief, organ functions
Inside of the nose	Reproductive organs	Respiration, digestion, pain relief, organ functions
Lips	Inner organs	Shows general disposition and weaknesses
Teeth	Organs according to TCM acupuncture system	Organ and metabolic function
Tongue	Digestive organs, liver, gallbladder, pancreas	The digestive system and its functioning
Iliac crest	Lumbar spine	Pain relief, problems resulting from dislocations of lumbar spine

Reflexology System	Main Structures	Influences
Back	Connective tissue of the internal organs	Stress or fatigue of the internal organs
Front of the torso	Connective tissue of the internal organs	Getting in touch with emotions and feelings ("organ talk")
Dermatomes	Segmental structure of the nervous system and its connection to the skin	Organs and body structures associated with the levels of the spine
Sclerotomes	Segmental structure of the nervous system and its connections to the bones	Organs and body structures associated with the levels of the spine
Forearms and lower legs	Vertebral spine and organs	Pain relief, organ function
Hands	Physical and mental aspects of the organs	Pain relief, organ function
Feet	Holographic image of the body	Organ function concerning body and mind

2

......

Reflexology Systems

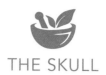

THE SKULL

Skull reflexology was introduced in 1978 in the context of acupuncture by Austrian physician Hans Zeitler. But acupuncture needles are not the only effective way to treat this area as reflexology massage provides an effective, noninvasive way to address a variety of disorders.

In this system of reflexology basically four areas can be treated, as follows:

1. Stripe for body sensation: for tingling, pain, phantom sensation
2. Stripe for muscle activity: for coordination and improvement in movement patterns

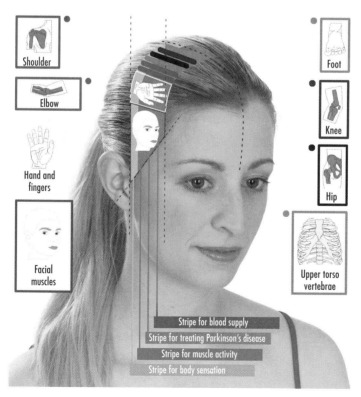

Shoulder

Elbow

Hand and fingers

Facial muscles

Foot

Knee

Hip

Upper torso vertebrae

Stripe for blood supply
Stripe for treating Parkinson's disease
Stripe for muscle activity
Stripe for body sensation

Reflexology on the skull

3. Stripe for Parkinson's disease: for movement and edema of the limbs

4. Stripe for blood supply: circulation and lymphatic activity

The most common indication for the use of the cranial reflexology is following a stroke, particularly when the person's ability to move is affected. By gently massaging the whole area of this reflexology system on the skull we have observed pronounced improvements in people even up to two years after the event, when medical guidelines say no further progress is possible.

Other applications of skull reflexology are related to problems of blood supply. Here self-massage brings relief for people who suffer from cold hands or feet. Just a little massage at the blood supply zone on the scalp for one or two minutes facilitates warmth in the affected limbs. For pain in the hands as a result of chronic rheumatic diseases we found that a soothing effect resulted from massaging the stripe associated with body sensation. Experience has shown that massaging the zone associated with Parkinson's disease with a crystal wand made out of rock crystal is beneficial, though the best effects are generally achieved with medical acupuncture. Finally, a rather unusual application concerns musicians. Whether for singing or for finger runs regular massage of all the skull zones brings an increase in musical skill and virtuosity.

While needle treatment requires precision application to one or more of the stripes on the skull, such precision is not necessary in reflexology massage. In fact it is even better to massage the area covering all four stripes. Be sure to adjust the intensity of the massage if there is any pain or discomfort in these areas.

The system illustrated on page 20 follows the coronal suture, the connective-tissue joint found between the frontal and the parietal bones of the skull. Through this system we can influence all the possible movement activities of the body.

About two-fifths of the cranium is involved in muscular functions.

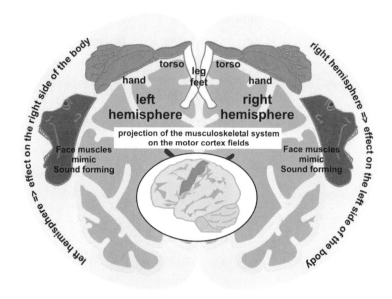

The cerebral cortex fields for movement in the brain

These include the facial expressions, sound shaping, and food intake. About one-fifth is occupied by the gripping, tactile, and fine motor functions of the hands, and the rest of the musculoskeletal system has to share the remaining two-fifths.

Tactile sensitivity in the fingers and our proprioception (the inner feeling of how our joints, ligaments, and muscles are stretched), motor function, nervous excitation, and vascular control—all these impulses on one side of the body are governed by the opposite hemisphere of the brain. The same principle applies in this reflexology system. For example, disorders of the right hand can be found on sensitive areas on the left side of the skull, and treatments of the zones of the shoulder on the right half of the skull will have their effects on the left shoulder.

THE OCCIPUT AND FOREHEAD

One important contribution to reflexology came from Japanese physician Toshikatsu Yamamoto, who among other things found a topography of the reflexology zones on the occiput and forehead. After more than twenty-five years of research Yamamoto published his findings in 1991, and they are now recognized worldwide.

The zone system of Yamamoto New Skull Acupuncture (YNSA) on the back of the head and the forehead aims mainly at the movement apparatus and the sense organs. Most reflexology systems achieve good results in functional ailments affecting movement and in conditions where diagnostic findings have led to unclear or contradictory conclusions. This is particularly true for Yamamoto's skull reflexology system.

Although YNSA describes the use of acupuncture needles, point reflexology massage with crystal wands and essential oils has proved to be very effective.

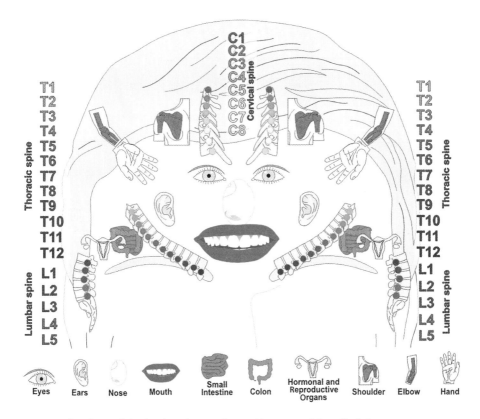

Reflexology of the forehead according to Yamamoto New Skull Acupuncture

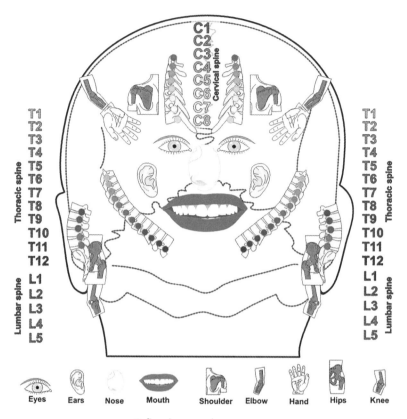

Reflexology on the occiput

The benefits of this reflexology system range from pain relief in the spinal column and joints to improvement in the capabilities of the sense organs. As well, our experience with this system has shown a positive influence on movement in general, including complex muscle-chain movement. This is especially applicable in cases of stroke, by supporting the affected area with regular gentle reflexology massage of both the forehead and the occiput.

THE NECK

A system of neck reflexology was first described in the 1950s by German orthopedist Karl Sell. Sell referred to the neck's "insertion

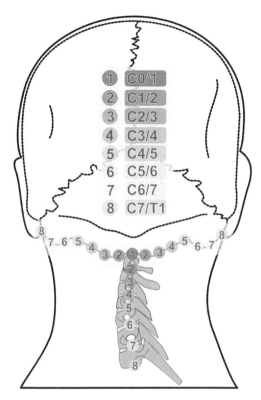

Reflexology points on the neck

zones" because at this area the muscles of the neck insert or attach to the back of the skull. Unfortunately neck reflexology has been largely unknown in most medical circles, although the system's zone delineations and convincing success have found new adherents in recent years.

This system can be used to deal with problems of the cervical spine, their nerve roots, and their areas of influence. Owing to the dense autonomic nervous system's cross-linking of the sympathetic, parasympathetic, and enteric nervous systems in the cervical spine there can often be a "distance effect," in which problems originating in the cervical area manifest in areas of the body that are distant from the spine, resulting in inexplicable physical symptoms and disorders.

As shown in the figure on page 24, all organs of the body are

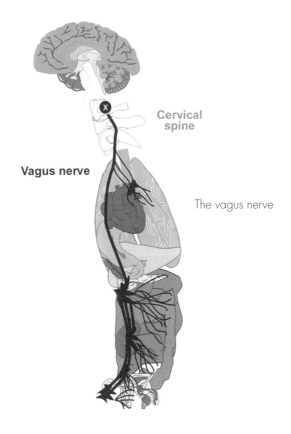

Cervical spine

Vagus nerve

The vagus nerve

supplied by the vagus nerve, the tenth cranial nerve that starts at the brain stem and travels all the way to the colon, making it the longest nerve of the autonomic nervous system. That is why disturbances in this upper area of the cervical spine are often associated with feeling nauseous and with digestive problems and troubles with the organs. This reflexology system is always worth a try to alleviate these symptoms as well as to treat neck contractions, whiplash, headache, spinal column–induced dizziness, or numb feelings of the hands and upper limbs—the list goes on and on. In treating this area soft circular point massage with the fingers or, even better, with the pointed end of a crystal wand, supported with essential oils, has proved effective.

Approximately 50 percent of the total flexion and extension of the cervical spine takes place in the first segment of the cervical spine. Here

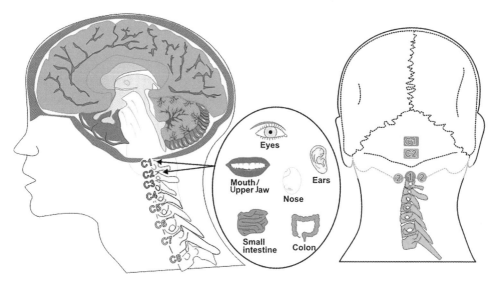

Reflexology points on the first and second segments of the cervical spine

there is a loop on the left and right vertebral arteries. From there these arteries, which are surrounded by a dense network of autonomic nerves, dive in to the head and are closely related to the inner ear. Treatment at the points served by the first segment of the cervical spine may be used to influence disorders in the movement of the head joints and to support treatment of brain-stem nerve problems, such as digestive irritations or a general feeling of malaise.

The second segment of the cervical spine is responsible for about 50 percent of the total rotation of the neck and is associated with movement of the head from side to side. Thus rotation of the head to the right is accompanied by a lateral inclination on the same side (and vice versa). Treatment at these reflexology points addresses disorders of the movement of the head and can alleviate toothaches in the upper jaw.

The third segment plays a major role in all movements of the lower cervical spine. Disturbances here result in difficulties in lifting the shoulders. This is the origination point of the phrenic nerve, the nerve that originates in the neck at C3-C5 and passes down

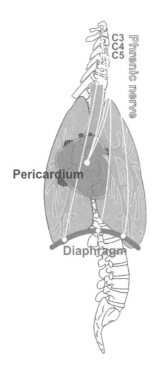

The phrenic nerve

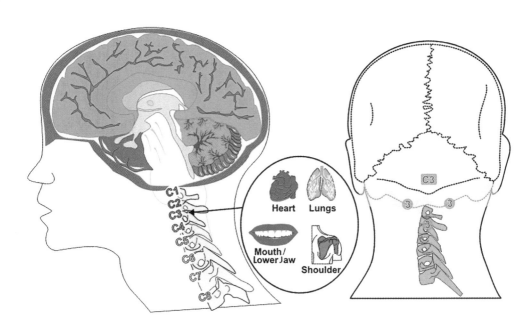

Reflexology points on the third segment of the cervical spine

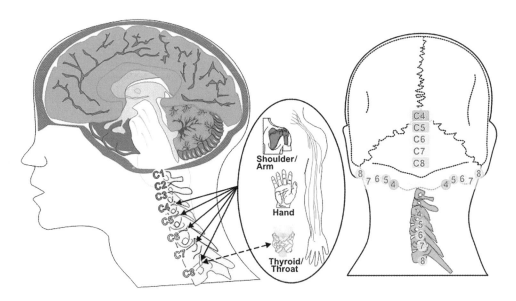

Reflexology points on the remaining segments of the cervical spine

between the lungs and heart to reach the diaphragm, supplying nervous impulses to the diaphragm and the pericardium. Treatment at these points can be effective for treating disorders of the cervical spine, such as deep-breathing problems or even heartbeat irregularities. Although gentle massage of all cervical segments has a positive effect on all kinds of nervous teeth problems (biting, chewing, gnashing), the second and third segments have the greatest influence on the teeth—the second segment on the teeth of the upper jaw and the third on the lower jaw.

The remaining segments of the cervical spine refer to the movements and sensitivity of the shoulders, arms, and hands. If there are tensions in the arm, such as from computer work (mouse elbow or typist's cramps), it will always be worth performing regular massages on these reflexology points on the neck. Additionally, massage of the reflexology points on these segments increases lymphatic flow in the throat, and those on the seventh and eighth segments can help regulate the thyroid gland.

THE LYMPHATIC NECK POINTS

Most head and neck problems are associated with disorders of the lymphatic drainage system. This includes headache, sore throat, stiff neck, irritations of the trigeminal nerve (which may result in toothache, facial tics, or even alterations of the dentition), and sinusitis. Eliminating lymph congestion often alleviates pain and tension.

The lymphatic belt is situated between the midpoints of the clavicles, front and back, somewhat like a necklace. Gentle massage of the points in this area will facilitate lymphatic drainage.

The points located on the transverse processes of the cervical spine are particularly suited for targeting lymph flow.

Gentle massage of the points on the left and right of the first cervical spine have proved particularly effective in the treatment of the nasal sinuses, promoting lymphatic drainage in this area. The points at the second cervical spine target problems of the upper jaw and the upper row of teeth. There, massages can help relieve pain after dental work. The same applies to the third cervical spine, which governs the teeth along the lower jaw. The tonsils and oral mucous membranes offer immune defense in the mouth and throat; the points at the fourth cervical spine support this system and help to reduce possible tension. Treating the points at the seventh cervical spine may alleviate irritations in connection with the ears.

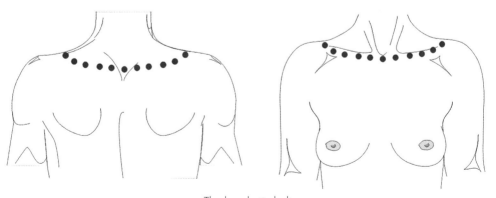

The lymphatic belt

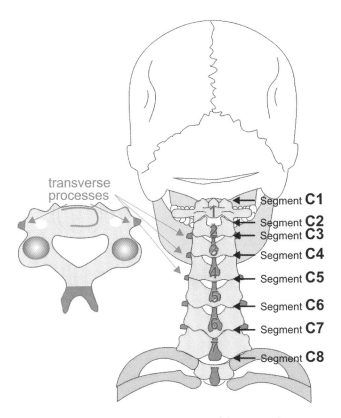

Transverse processes of the cervical spine

All massages in the neck should be very gentle, without any pain, as pain has the reverse effect of increasing problems. Quite often it is sufficient to simply touch these points with a finger in place for a few moments until you sense a release of tension under the finger.

THE FACE

One would think that the face would be completely familiar from shaving or doing one's makeup or hair, and yet we use only a fraction of the information it provides. The facial expression gives us insight into the personality of a person, since it mostly works unconsciously and is to a great extent directly linked to dopamine, the hormone responsible for

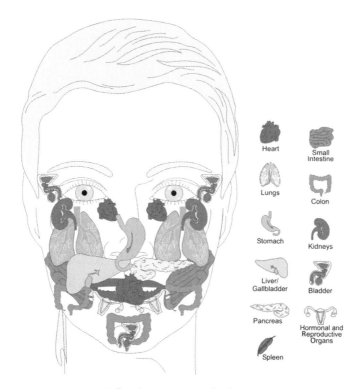

Heart

Small Intestine

Lungs

Colon

Stomach

Kidneys

Liver/ Gallbladder

Bladder

Pancreas

Hormonal and Reproductive Organs

Spleen

Reflexology areas on the face

our moods. All emotions are clearly recognizable in the face, whether fear, worry, anger, sadness, pleasure, or joy. The changing expressions of the face bring a sense of aliveness to one's appearance, but when an emotion becomes frozen on the face, becoming a constant feature, it is an indication that the energy flow in the body is disturbed, and an organ system is receiving either too much or not enough energy. This is when reflexology can be valuable.

Traditional Chinese medicine describes the connection between the emotions and the organs. An excess of anger or fear will show up as a permanent state of emotional strain on the face. For example, a deep fold from the left angle of the mouth to the nasal margin points to problems with the pancreas as a result of a chronic lack of joy and an insatiable thirst for recognition. The pancreas will then be susceptible to weakness as reflected in all kinds of diseases. Whether a person has

Elements / Analogues	Wood	Fire	Earth	Metal	Water
Climatic influence	Wind	Heat	Humidity	Dryness	Cold
Color	Green	Red	Yellow	White	Black
Organ YIN / YANG	Liver Gallbladder	Heart Small Intestine	Spleen/Pancreas Stomach	Lungs Colon	Kidneys Bladder
Tissue	Muscles	Vessels	Connective Tissue	Skin	Bones
Emotions − / +	Rage / Anger / Purposefulness	Exuberance / Joy	Sorrows / Contemplation	Coldness / Mourning	Anxiety / Fear / Confidence

TCM links the five elements to the physical, mental, and emotional components of a human being.

the flu or is involved in an accident, when the body activates the repair brigades, quotas must be deducted from the organ in question, and the strain shows up in the face.

When information reaches the unconscious parts of the brain they work as a sorting center for our perceptions. A 1996 issue of *Newsweek* magazine titled "The Biology of Beauty" pointed out that we are born with an idea about what male and female attractiveness consists of. In males a prominent chin, which is deemed attractive, is formed by a genetically high level of testosterone. However high testosterone levels weaken the immune system, so while a man with a prominent chin is considered a good mating partner who can support and defend his family, he may fall victim to his aggressiveness and develop various health issues as a result. Females are mostly influenced by estrogen. A high level of estrogen results in a round, symmetrical face that is a female standard of beauty, one that indicates the probability that pregnancy will be easy and without complications. Even when these basic patterns remain in our unconscious mind the social implications for our species go back as far as the Stone Age.

The reflexology areas on the face react very well to gentle, soft massage techniques. There is almost nothing as relaxing and soothing as a facial massage. At the same time, the associated organ functions are strengthened. Cosmetologists have been aware of this effect for a long time, although they may not be aware of the equally positive effects on the organs that their facial massages provide.

When massaging the face you can increase the beneficial effects by incorporating essential oils. But the best therapy of all is laughter—it loosens up all the structures and muscles in the face, strengthens the heart-lung system, and provides the body cells with fresh oxygen. Thus laughter and cheerfulness enhance any healing process.

THE IRIS OF THE EYES

Since 1873, when Ignaz von Peczely published his systematic topographical assignments of the organs to the iris, iridology has become a

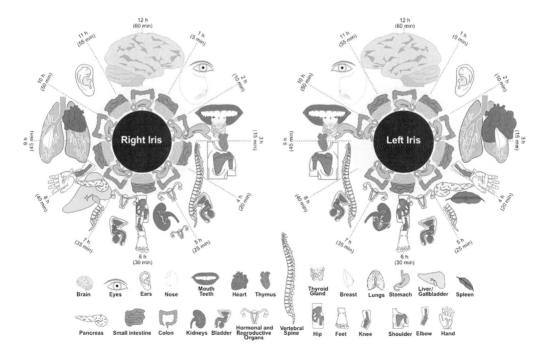

Iridology, a system of reflexology in the iris of the eyes

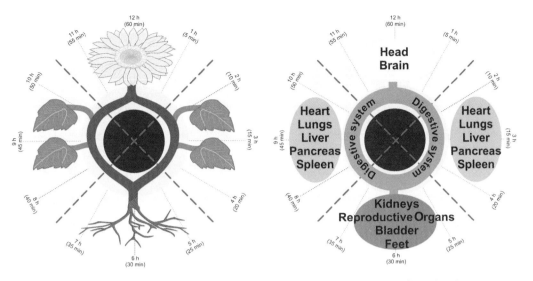

The human being as a plant in the eye   Organ structure as reflected in the eye

widely accepted modality in natural healing. Through the iris we can observe the body-mind matrix and diagnose everything from organ-related disorders to mental, emotional, and even spiritual imbalances.

Iridology evaluates the iris according to different criteria that allow us to recognize a predisposition for certain problems. These include asthma, allergies, eczema, and diabetes. In acute as well as chronic diseases, certain signs occur in the iris that are mostly indications of weakness appearing in the form of cavities, cloudy or darkened areas in the iris, colored spots, or pigments. In addition the formation of conspicuous vascular drawings that refer to certain organs can be observed on the whites of the eyes. A trained iris diagnostician can recognize in just a few moments indications of certain problems or organ weaknesses. This can lead to further diagnostic assessments. Iridology also indicates the quality of the function of the autonomic nervous system, particularly the impulses of the sympathetic nervous system. Long before a problem manifests in an organ it can show up in the eyes.

The structure of the iris resembles that of a flower, including roots, stem, and blossom, as shown above.

Here the blossom symbolizes the head with all its functions comprising the brain for controlling conscious and unconscious processes. Within the frill of the iris we find the stem, which corresponds to the digestive system, from the esophagus to the rectum. This is followed by the roots, which represent the kidneys, the organs of the abdomen, the legs and feet. Finally the leaves symbolize our organs of substance intake, transport, and processing: lungs, heart, liver, spleen, and pancreas. The fascinating design of this reflexology system in the iris offers a multidimensional structure that can provide the basis for early interventions to maintain or to regain health.

THE EARS

Reflexology of the ear, or ear acupuncture, is also known as *auriculotherapy,* in reference to the outer portion of the ear, the auricle. Like all other forms of reflexology it is premised on the fact that the auricle is a micro system that reflects the entire body. Auriculotherapy was first proposed by French neurologist Paul Nogier in his 1957 "Treatise of Auriculotherapy." Nogier conducted a number of clinical trials based on a phrenological method of projection of a fetal homunculus (a human in miniature) on the ear to reference certain physical complaints and the corresponding points for treatment.

The facing figure shows that the auricle resembles an embryo whose head lies in the earlobe. There are no coincidences in the body, especially not in its forms, thus the embryo shape of the ear points to the time of human gestation, the most active period in human life. That is why the main contraindication of ear reflexology is during pregnancy, since the stimuli can lead to unintended tension in the growing fetus.

Ear reflexology works something like a switchboard. When there is a disturbance in the stomach or the heart the affected organ calls the switchboard, at which point a signal light turns on in the corresponding reflexology zone of the auricle assigned to that organ. This signal may be a sore spot or an irritation. Reflexology treatment at that point

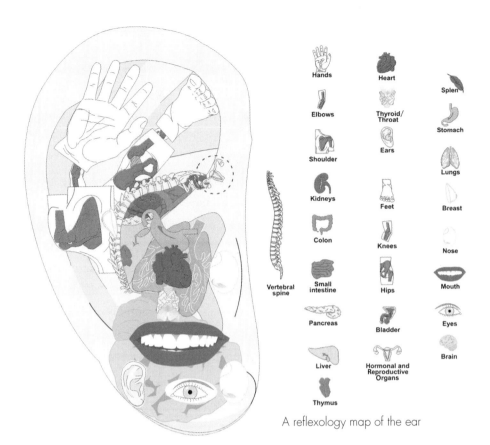

Hands	Heart	Spleen
Elbows	Thyroid/Throat	Stomach
Shoulder	Ears	Lungs
Kidneys	Feet	Breast
Colon	Knees	Nose
Vertebral spine	Small intestine	Hips	Mouth
Pancreas	Bladder	Eyes
Liver	Hormonal and Reproductive Organs	Brain
Thymus		

A reflexology map of the ear

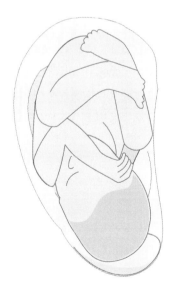

A fetal homunculus projected onto the auricle of an ear

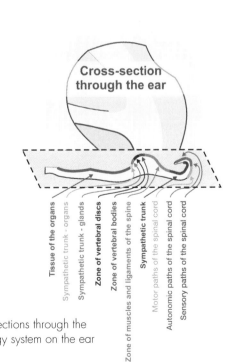

Cross-section through the ear

Tissue of the organs
Sympathetic trunk - organs
Sympathetic trunk - glands
Zone of vertebral discs
Zone of vertebral bodies
Zone of muscles and ligaments of the spine
Sympathetic trunk
Motor paths of the spinal cord
Autonomic paths of the spinal cord
Sensory paths of the spinal cord

Cross-sections through the reflexology system on the ear

or points serves as a connection to the maintenance unit, which works quickly to address the situation. This means that on the physical level we often achieve pain relief with ear reflexology in moments, and on the mental and emotional levels the effects on depression, smoking cessation, and weight issues are quite impressive.

It is almost unimaginable that there is so much to be found on such a small surface, the auricle of the ear. The main diagnostic methods for determining which points to address are muscle testing, pulse testing, or electronic point testing (methods described in the next part of this book). In treating ears acupuncture needles are used, sometimes in combination with a laser or with electrical impulses. But we have found that reflexology using the pointed end of a crystal wand is equally effective.

A frequent question is "Which ear should be treated?" and another is "Does the point require activation or dissipation?" The answers to these questions can be found through the various testing methods described in the next part of this book, but for the first question we found that on the side of the body where the disorder is present the reflexology zones react more intensely. Nevertheless it has proved beneficial to treat both ears as this way disturbances disappear considerably faster.

One comment on piercings: Without a doubt most people who get their ears pierced do not test to see if the piercing occurs at a system-relevant point. This is a more significant issue in the case of multiple piercings on an ear, which can cause far-reaching consequences for the autonomic nervous system. For this reason I advise against multiple piercings.

THE BRIDGE OF THE NOSE

The skin on the outside of the sense organs of the head have special reflexology qualities. It seems that these areas are more sensitive to outside impulses. Even if the auricles of the ears are the most familiar of the reflexology systems of the sense organs, the nasal bridge can also be used for treatment. There are two different approaches to

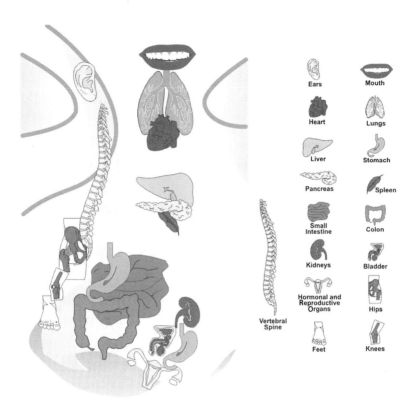

The nasal therapy system of reflexology on the bridge of the nose

The naso-labial system of reflexology
on the bridge of the nose

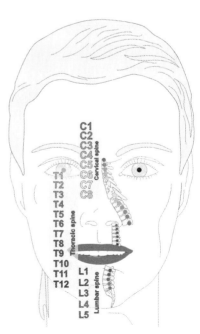

this form of reflexology. One of them, the nasal therapy system, follows some additional points found in traditional Chinese medicine. The other one, the naso-labial system, was discovered in 1990 by the president of the Russian Association of Acupuncture and Traditional Medicine, Dr. Alexander Kachan.

The nasal therapy system has in its topography three lines, where the organs are in the middle line and to the left and to the right, and the movement apparatus has its spots. The naso-labial system shows another system. Here the points of the vertebral spine and the limbs seem to be arranged like a cord of beads. The cervical spine is situated along the nostrils, the thoracic spine follows between the nose and the lips, and the lumbar spine has points under the lip on the chin. As for the extremities, the shoulders and elbows are found above the upper canines, and the hips and the knees have reflexology points above the lower canines.

Though acupuncture needle applications are the most effective way to treat in either of these systems, reflexology massage, particularly with the pointed end of a crystal wand or a cotton swab soaked with diluted essential oil, can be very effective in improving functional symptoms of the associated organs and painful conditions of the musculoskeletal system. These massages should always be carried out very gently. It should be noted that these reflexology zones have significance in face diagnosis because they indicate which organ is exposed to stress at the moment. For this reason pimples, impure skin, or recurring skin disorders on the bridge of the nose are clear signs of an imbalance in the body.

THE INSIDE OF THE NOSE

The zones in the interior of the nose were first discovered in 1883 by Rudolph Voltolini, a German-Polish physician. Ten years later Wilhelm Fliess, a German otolaryngologist and friend and collaborator of Sigmund Freud, elucidated his theory of "nasal reflex neurosis," which postulated the connection between the nose and the genitals. Notably, Fliess used cocaine base in the zones inside the nose to treat female disorders of the reproductive organs, purportedly to great success. He also played an important part in the development of Freud's method of psychoanalysis.

Along the nasal turbinates in the nose four zones are clearly related to the autonomic nervous system. These zones range from the reproductive organs, digestion, and breathing to the regulation of the head functions. The main targets of this reflexology system, however, are issues involving the female and male sexual organs.

Self-treatment of points on the inside of the nose can help women with any disturbances of the menstrual cycle and with symptoms of menopause; in men, self-treatment inside the nose in these

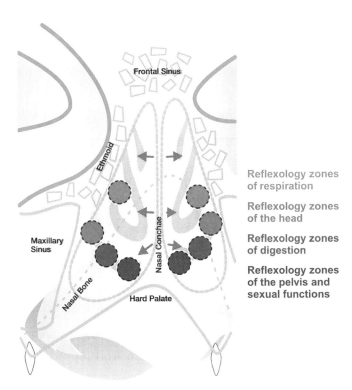

A reflexology map inside the nose

zones benefit those with prostate problems. The relevant zones are clearly detectable as sensitive areas inside the nose. The technique is quite easy: Two cotton swabs are soaked with diluted essential oil; then, very gently, the zones are *simultaneously* massaged in both nostrils, just behind the nostrils. For women lavender or rose essential oil is recommended; for men sandalwood oil has proved suitable. The zones should be massaged very gently and without pain for about one or two minutes three to five times a day.

The other reflexology zones inside the nose are reserved for medical use only. For this purpose, long cotton swabs (about 15 cm, or 6 inches) are soaked with diluted essential oil and gently pushed along the nasal turbinates to the zonal areas. The oils for these therapeutic applications should be chosen by testing. The soaked swabs can stay on the zonal areas for between five and fifteen minutes. This method exerts very intense stimuli to the autonomic nervous system, so for this reason care must be taken to be extremely careful and gentle. The effects are quite impressive. Alleviation of spastic bronchitis, asthma, and mucous membrane swelling can be achieved in the respiratory tract. By treating the gastrointestinal system zone the liver, pancreas, and GALT (gut-associated lymphoid tissue) can be supported. The GALT is in control of the entire defense functions of the immune system. This explains why treatments in these zones inside the nose have proved to be effective in addressing allergies and immunodeficiency disorders. Concerning the functions of the head, the applications cover a range of indications, including control of vascular tension in the brain, headache, and migraine.

Even when the medical applications of this form of reflexology are out of reach for most people the applications that address any kind of disturbance in the male or female reproductive organs are quite accessible to anyone and have proved to be successful for more than a hundred years.

THE LIPS

The lips have a reflexology system that dates back to their use by ancient ayurvedic physicians. Certain signs on the lips are also well known to us. These cosmetic defects or annoying irritations include slight pigment changes, small mucous defects, or herpes vesicles that usually show up again and again in the same place. People often try to deal with these signs with cosmetic measures, usually in vain since these signs point to weaknesses in the body. They will return until the affected organ or system is treated with suitable methods. Then the signs will no longer appear.

One of the most obvious signs on the lips is displayed on the rim of the lower lip. A swelling there indicates overactivity of the reproductive organs, particularly the female uterus or the male prostate gland. In women this is a symptom of a disorder in the menstruation cycle, and in men it is a sign of an irritation of the prostate. Another sign of imbalance we often find on the lips are mucous irritations in the zones of the lungs, which indicate that the immune system is stressed by bronchial problems.

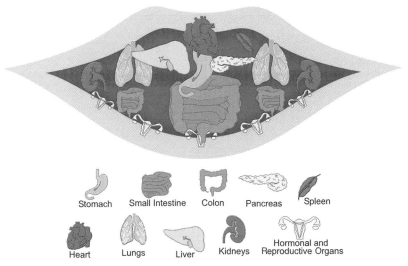

A reflexology map of the lips

THE TEETH

The assignment of the organs and body structures to the teeth were described in 1968 by German holistic dentist and medical doctor Reinhold Voll, one of the pioneers of electro-acupuncture. The assignment of the teeth to the organs closely follows the five elements system of traditional Chinese medicine, with the main organ issues related to this system.

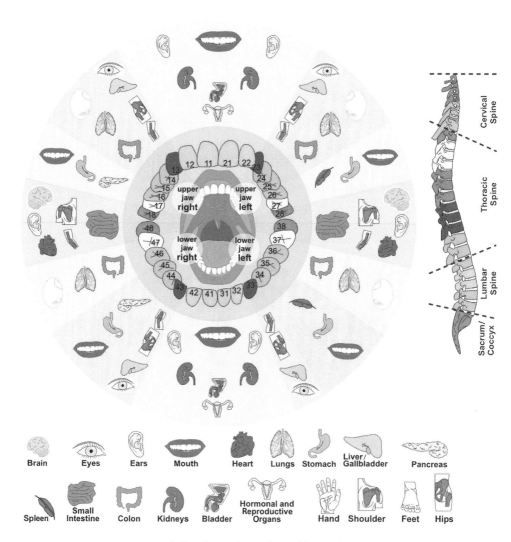

Reflexology relationships of the teeth

The incisors have a special relationship to the kidneys and bladder and to urogenital problems, disorders of hormonal regulation, impotence, and loss of libido. Additionally these teeth relate to neuralgia, headache, tinnitus, and chronic tonsillitis.

The canines are related to liver and gallbladder issues, including bile complaints, digestive problems, disturbances of the metabolic function, and inadequate detoxification of the organism with general fatigue. Also, eye problems, glaucoma, cataract, headache, migraine, hip and knee problems, blockages of the sacroiliac joint, and sciatica are problems that correspond to the canines.

The molars are associated with lung, colon, spleen, pancreas, and stomach problems. Gastrointestinal complaints, heartburn, bronchitis, asthma, colds with inflammation of the upper airways, allergies, diabetic disposition, nasal sinus infections, and shoulder and arm problems are some of the symptoms.

Holistic dentists know that quite often after the wisdom teeth are removed heart complaints, blood-pressure fluctuations, or tinnitus disappear. These teeth are also responsible for intestinal problems, unusual sensations in the hands, and disorders of the nervous system.

THE TONGUE

Almost everyone, since childhood, has heard a doctor say, "Stick out your tongue." The purpose of tongue diagnosis is to study the surface of the tongue, which describes a person's state of health. A yellowish tongue indicates liver problems, a brownish covering is evidence of intestinal troubles, and whitish pads are signs of stomach problems. But the tongue has a much wider range of diagnostic possibilities since it represents a map of the entire digestive system and its functions. This was systematized in 1957 by Anton Strobl, a German physician. Reflexology on the tongue is less devoted to the quality of the coating and more to structural signs. These can be red spots

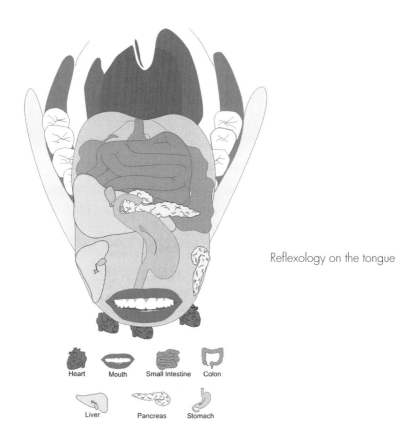

Reflexology on the tongue

Heart   Mouth   Small Intestine   Colon

Liver   Pancreas   Stomach

or swellings as signs of intestinal inflammation or incisions as an indication that an organ suffers from a loss of energy.

The organs have their corresponding reflexology zones on the tongue on the same side as in the body. On the right side of the tongue are the zones for the liver and gallbladder, the duodenum, and the ascending colon. On the left are the pancreas and spleen as well as the descending colon, and along the middle of the tongue are mainly the stomach and the small intestine. Under the tip of the tongue we find the reflexology zones of the heart. Cardiovascular problems manifest as inflammations around the tip of the tongue. When the veins are prominent on the underside of the tongue or when the tongue is slightly bluish it indicates heart problems, which are often caused by congestion in the digestive system, since the stomach and the heart are in close proximity in the body. In overweight persons the digestive organs are pressed against the pericardial sac and so they diminish the space of the heart. If there are heart complaints when lying on the left side they are usually the result of too rich a diet; these complaints usually disappear soon after a reasonable dietary change.

Tongue reflexology is mainly a diagnostic system; even if we can recognize various malfunctions as signs showing up on the tongue, treatment on the tongue itself is limited. The only effective tongue treatment we know of is the scraping of the tongue as a daily morning cleansing ritual, an ayurvedic practice that is a very effective way to treat the entire digestive system.

THE BACK

In dealing with our changing environment and its many stresses we are constantly brought to our limits. And once the body exceeds its limits it comes into a chronic state of stress. If we are chronically overloaded the body will force us, one way or another, to rest. Whereas a single organ under stress sends warning signals to its corresponding reflexology zones, the back will still perform its duties however best it can. Each organ has about three times its normal capacity as a reserve, thus ensuring survival. But with compound stresses the signs begin to show up as back problems.

Reflexology on the back indicates how far organ systems are stressed beyond their capacities. Back reflexology coincides closely with the Shu points of traditional Chinese medicine (TCM). These twelve "transporting points" are associated with each of the twelve organs and are supplied by specific corresponding dorsal and ventral nerves coming out the spine. They are located on the Bladder meridian on the back, and in TCM they serve as points for both diagnosis and treatment. The earliest masters of TCM who lived several thousand years ago found these points, which lie mostly in the spinal segments of the organs.

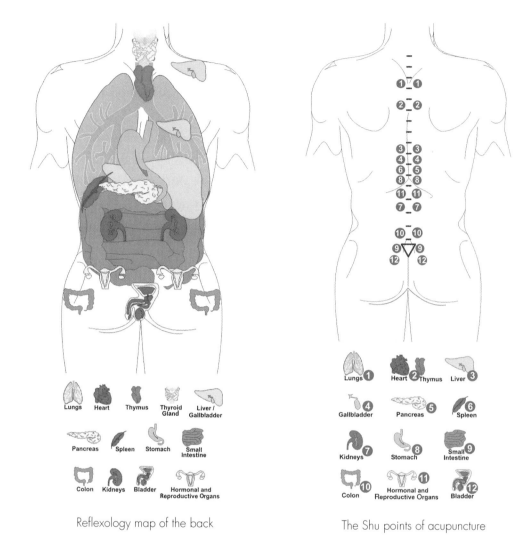

Reflexology map of the back

The Shu points of acupuncture

For example, in the case of swelling of a skin area or pimples on the back, this is a sign that other warning signals have already been passed. The autonomic nervous system is reacting with an irritation and an overstimulation both in the affected organ as well as in the corresponding reflexology zone on the back. If the organ becomes chronically overloaded it withdraws energetically. The reflexology zones will show this quite literally by displaying a retrieving of the skin. Opposite to a swelling, the retrieving feels harder and denser than the surrounding tissue when palpated, and the skin in the area sometimes feels dry. This is a sign that the associated organ has reduced its activities to a minimum. The condition can be influenced positively with greater awareness of the problem and with reflexology massages. This direct contact with the skin is still one of the most effective methods of treatment. To supplement reflexology back massage use gel packs, herbal pads, and essential oils. For best results the packs and pads should be applied with a temperature at about 105–110°F. Even if the problems cannot be remedied with back treatments the various applications will help alleviate pain. To address the condition long-term we should remember the order of priorities for healing as described in the Huangdi Neijing, a 2,500-year-old Chinese medical text regarded as a source of TCM:

1. Right life, mental hygiene, and exercise
2. Right nutrition
3. Medicines and herbal teas
4. Acupuncture reflexology treatment

THE FRONT OF THE TORSO

The reflexology zones on the front of the torso follow in their organization the same position of the organs in the body. So the zones of the lungs and the heart are to be found in the thoracic region, the zones of the digestive organs and the kidneys are on the belly, and the zones of the urinary tract and sexual organs are on the abdomen. In addition to signs of organic disturbances, the front of the torso holds the protected area of the feelings and emotions.

The reflexology points on the front of the torso correspond to the Mu points of TCM. These twelve points on the chest and abdomen are the "gathering points" of their associated organs. In reflexology as in acupuncture they are used to release congestion or tonify weak energy conditions in the associated organs for overall well-being.

The Mu points also offer a map of the emotions and play a

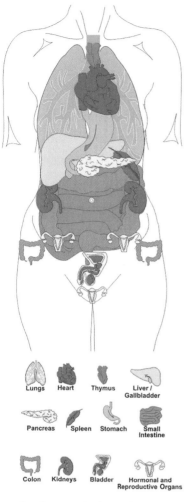

Reflexology on the front of the torso

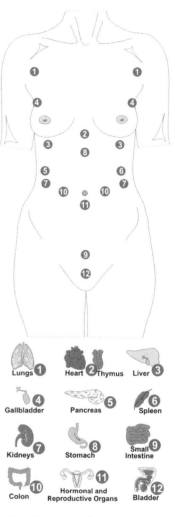

The Mu points of acupuncture
on the front of the torso

prominent role on the psychosomatic level because they address the enteric nervous system, which is responsible not only for the digestion of food but for the emotions as well. Some common expressions give us an idea of the deeper meanings contained within these important points. Whether we suffer from a "broken heart," when fear is felt "in the pit of the stomach," or if we have to "swallow our pride," our words point to how our emotions affect the organ concerned. This reflexology system is thus enormously valuable beyond the purely physical level for revealing inner conflicts that would otherwise lead to physical disturbances if not resolved.

When we bury unresolved feelings in the depths of the unconscious they often show up as skin problems on the front of the torso, therefore treatment here aims at a better understanding of one's feelings—feelings that are connected to specific organs. For example, besides any medical association it has, a patch of rough skin or eczema in the zone of the lungs might be saying "What do the lungs want to tell me?" "Do I really need to yell at someone?" or "Does something take my breath away?" It is not important whether we are actually coughing or whether we are restricted in our breathing; the issue targets the emotions or feelings we associate with the appearance of a disturbance on the skin at this location. In this way reflexology offers insight into the mind-body connection, allowing us to address the deep, underlying emotional causes of a problem.

A simple technique for resolving conflicted emotions as displayed on the upper front of the torso, the balloon visualization, is found in part 4 of this book. Other methods that target the emotions are Rolfing, Postural Integration, and Rebalancing. Our inner voice always gives us the right answers, even if they are sometimes surprising.

DERMATOMES, SCLEROTOMES, AND MYOTOMES

These anatomical terms refer to the embryonic development of the skin and movement systems of the body. At about the twentieth day after conception the first pair of somites appear, the forerunner of our vertebral segments. This first segment of our vertebral spine will later become the occiput. By the thirty-fifth day we have forty-four pairs of somites. At the sixtieth day that number is reduced to the final number of between thirty-two and thirty-five somites (the reduction is due to the coccyx, which may have more or less ossi-fied vertebrae). From these somites the dermatomes, sclerotomes, and myotomes emigrate with the growth of the fetus. Until the ninth week of pregnancy, the dermatomes, sclerotomes, and myotomes are together; after that they begin to differentiate. From the tenth week on the dermatomes organize into the skin structures, the sclerotomes become the bone structures, and the myotomes the muscle structures. The nerves accompany this growth development to supply the different structures.

The discovery of dermatomes in 1893 by British physicians Henry Head and Stephen McKenzie was one of the first great achievements of modern neurology, a discovery that explained the segmental structure of the peripheral nervous system and its connections to the skin. It took nearly thirty more years until these discoveries were used in practice when in 1925 the German physician Ferdinand Huneke injected the anesthetic drug Novocain (procaine) into the dermatomes in a method he called neural therapy. This application is still successfully used to regulate the autonomous nervous system and improve organ function. Injections of procaine, or more recently lidocaine, can produce inexplicable far-reaching effects, particularly in cases where there is a scar in the reflexology zone. A neural therapy injection into such a scar can relieve pain in a completely different area of the body, liberate restricted movements, and stimulate organ function. Early in my career I treated a seventy-five-year-old patient with scars from wounds he suffered in World War II. As I injected 0.1 milliliter of procaine into a scar on his lower back he began to cry in joy—he could lift his right arm for the first time in sixty years.

A few years after Huneke's neural therapy breakthrough, in 1929, physiotherapist Elizabeth Dicke developed a plowlike massage characterized by a pulling technique through the dermatomes, the connective-tissue massage (how she made this discovery is described in part 1 of this book).

After Head and McKenzie described the dermatomes, researchers started looking for the other tissues that followed a particular

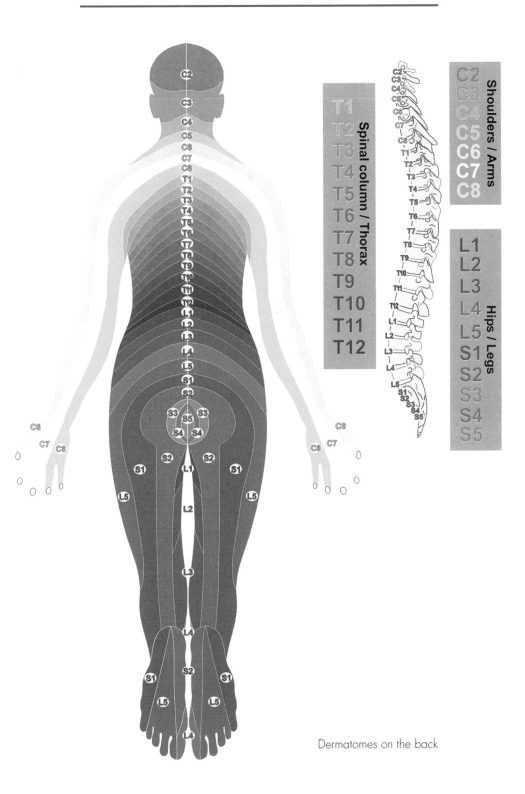

Dermatomes on the back

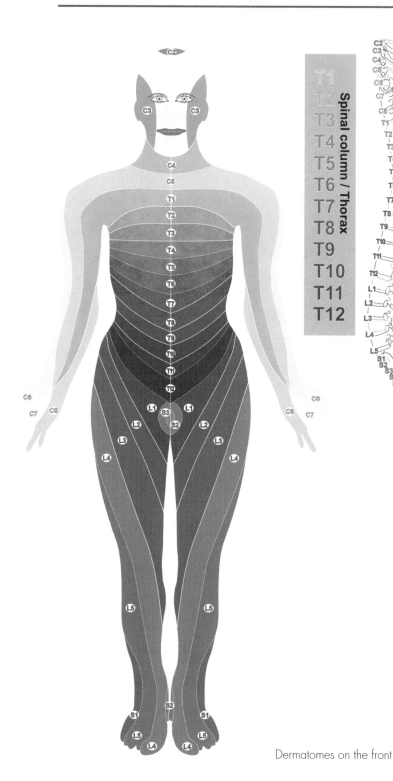

Dermatomes on the front

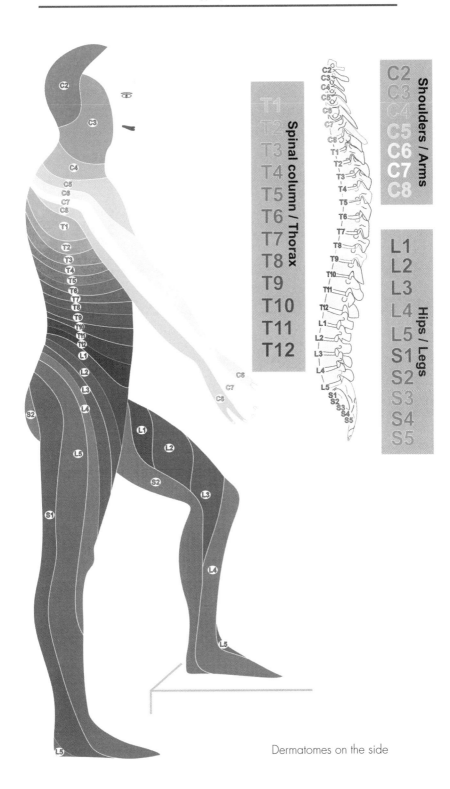

Dermatomes on the side

organizational pattern. In 1944, American orthopedists Verne Inman and John Saunders found these on the bones. The *sclerotomes,* as they called these zones on the bones and the skin of the bones, are pain- or contact-sensitive regions on the skeletal system that follow a disturbed nerve root and its area of influence. As a spin-off of the discovery of the sclerotomes, around the same time researchers found the segmental assignments of the muscles to the nerves of the respec-

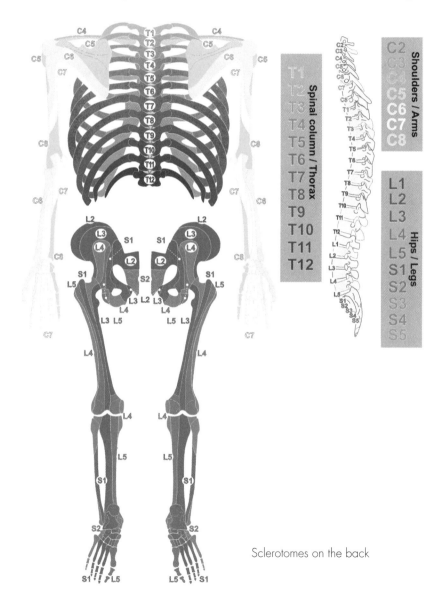

Sclerotomes on the back

tive segment in the vertebral column and called these *myotomes.*

These connections of the muscles go beyond neurology. As with the Mu points of traditional Chinese medicine, the muscles on the front of the body govern the emotions and can therefore be used to release stress patterns and traumatic experiences. In addition to reflexology, methods that use the muscles for emotional release include Rolfing, Postural Integration, and Rebalancing. Kinesiology shows

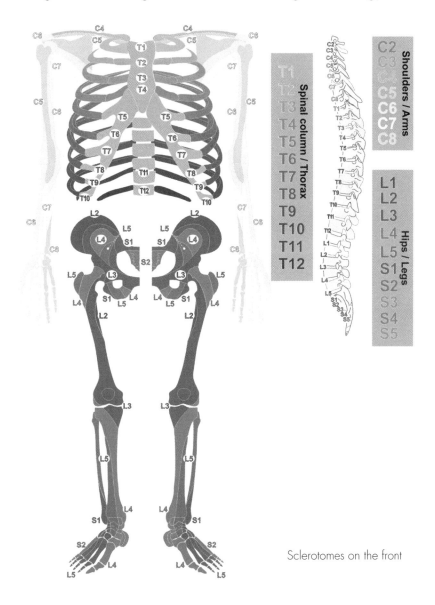

Sclerotomes on the front

that there is a connection between the muscles and muscle groups and certain organ functions as delineated by traditional Chinese medicine, such that we know which muscles are associated with which organs. For example, the stomach muscles and those of the

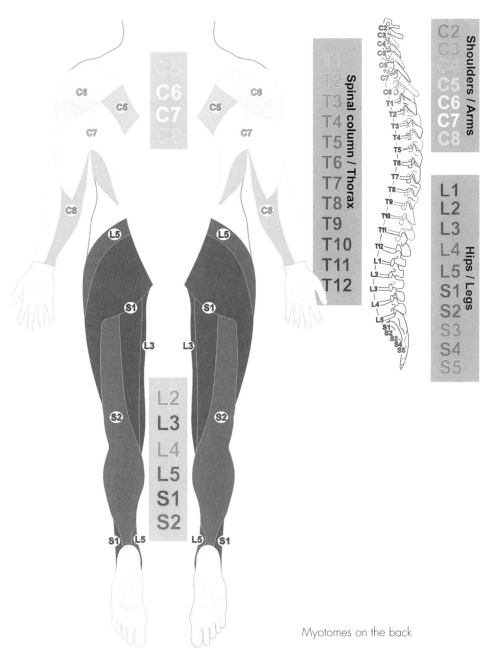

Myotomes on the back

upper thigh refer to the small intestine, the latissimus muscle on the back is associated with the pancreas, and the diaphragm corresponds with the lungs. Another consideration involves the complex patterns of synergistic and antagonistic muscles that every movement follows.

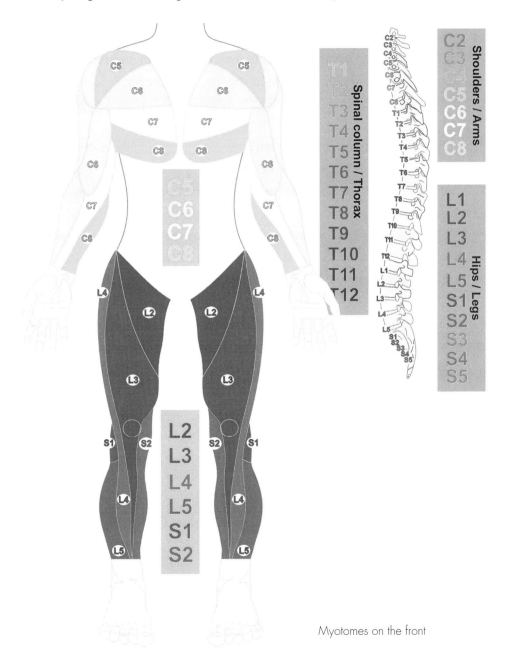

Myotomes on the front

Disorders in these patterns lead to inefficient movements that require a high expenditure of energy, resulting in painful muscular trigger points.

The more efficiently we perform movements the less energy we will need to do so. T'ai chi, qigong, and martial arts practitioners follow this principle, which is why most of their movements are diagonal patterns. For example, a bending of the left leg corresponds to a similar movement of the right arm, while at the same time the right leg and left arm are extended. We find this principle in the physio-therapeutic technique of Proprioceptive Neuromuscular Facilitation (PNF), which aims at rehabilitating and stretching muscles to get at maximal movement results. In this technique certain muscle groups are stretched while the muscles performing the opposite function contract. This is an example of the diagonal pattern of movement that greatly helps stroke patients or those who have broken a bone and are trying to regain their movement abilities.

The nerve connections of the organs to the dermatomes, sclerotomes, and myotomes are organized in segments; each nerve connection emerges between two vertebrae. These spinal segments are connected to two high-speed links of information. One of them, the spinal cord, is responsible for outbound movement impulses and inbound sensations. The other route, the sympathetic trunk, consists of two chains running along the front side of the spine, providing impulses for the regulation of the organs. Each floor—the area defined by a vertebral segment—has connections to these two expressways. In fact these are similar to highway junctions from which other roads branching off the highway begin. From the sympathetic chain the impulses go to organs, vessels, and to the skin, while the nerve fibers from the spinal cord lead directly to the muscles, to the sensory systems, and to the structures of the spine itself. The illustration on page 59 shows these connections in the example of breathing.

Connective-tissue massage in the dermatomes requires special training, but every other kind of massage has a beneficial effect on the connective tissue as well. Incorporating diluted essential oils or crystals can really enhance massage in the dermatomes.

Another method of treating the dermatomes is the wrap, as in the liver wrap, in which cooked potatoes are wrapped in a damp, warm cloth. The potatoes must not be too warm because they could cause scalding. This wrap is put on the area under the right rib cage where the liver is located for about half an hour. In this way the liver is activated via the dermatomes for a better metabolism and detoxification of the whole body. If bile stones have been diagnosed, one should consult a physician before this treatment, because if the stones are large,

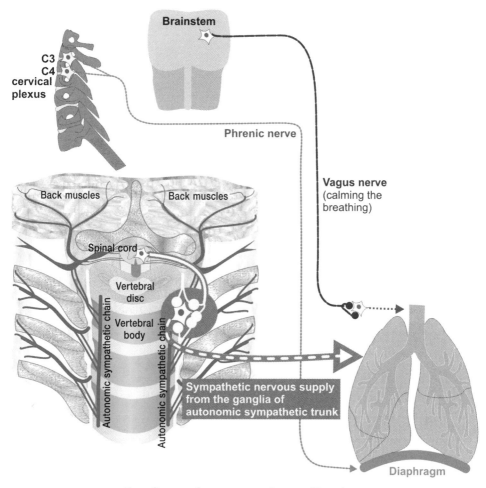

The influence of a segment in the act of breathing

cramping could result. A wrap can be applied to any of the dermatomes for an effect on the associated organs or body structures. (It can also be used on the lower abdomen to relieve discomfort during menstruation, on the knees for soothing arthritis pain, and on the chest in cases of bronchitis.)

The sclerotomes are mainly used for diagnostic purposes, since a form of massage on the skin of the bones that was developed in the 1950s turned out to be very painful and disappeared from the treatment catalog. To date we have only a fragmentary understanding of how to make use of the possibilities of the myotomes. Here physiotherapists have the most comprehensive knowledge of trigger points, trigger chains, and movement patterns.

THE ILIAC CREST

The lumbar vertebral column, in particular the segment between the fifth lumbar vertebra and the lumbosacral transitional vertebra, is among the most vulnerable points in the human body. Research over the past twenty-five years points to the interplay between static elements such as vertebrae and intervertebral discs and dynamic elements such as ligaments and muscles. This is complemented by a sophisticated software that controls the neurological muscle chains, equilibrium reactions, and different nervous-system responses of the body. This explains why quite often problems with the bladder or with the reproductive organs, for example, are associated with a misalignment of the lumbar vertebrae. Sometimes one's sex life improves once the lumbar spine is realigned properly.

Metabolic, psychosomatic, and energetic influences are important for the free flow of energies within our body. This is true in a special way for the spinal column. Reflexology has the potential to maintain the flow of nervous impulses, discharge metabolic wastes, and improve posture. In the 1950s orthopedist Karl Sell found on the iliac crest an equivalent to the lymphatic belt located at the cervical

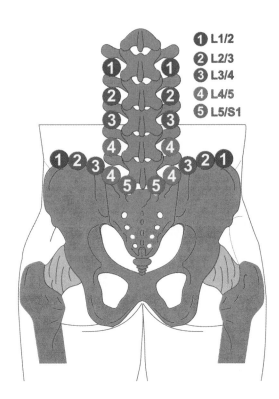

1 L1/2
2 L2/3
3 L3/4
4 L4/5
5 L5/S1

Reflexology zones on
the iliac crest

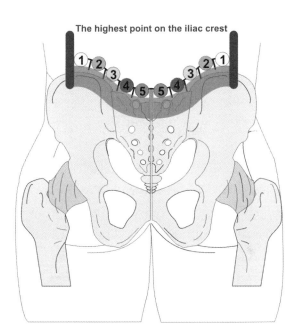

Finding the reflexology points
on the iliac crest

neckline. This system on the iliac crest is a complete reflexology system with points along the upper pelvic rim. These points show irritations of the lumbar spine and are very effective treatment locations for releasing pain.

To find the relevant points to treat a condition of back pain in the lumbar spine and its specific areas of influence the distance between the highest point of the pelvic rim and the farthest point on the back of the iliac crest are divided into five parts. The innermost fifth on the back corresponds to the fifth lumbar spine, and the outermost fifth on the front to the first lumbar spine. The remaining segments from the second to the fourth lumbar spine are distributed between them accordingly, as shown in the illustrations on page 61.

Looking at the different segments in the lumbar spine, L1 influences intestinal motility. Massages there can help alleviate constipation and diarrhea. Via L2 we may control the ileocecal valve between the small intestine and colon and lymphatic flow from the legs. L3 relates to the uterus and prostate and is helpful for menstruation problems and in male menopause. Additionally this segment is the main one for knee problems. L4 reaches to the ovaries and testicles and controls emptying of the bladder. L5 has a great influence on blood supply and lymphatic drainage of the lower limbs.

When there are disturbances in the spine we will find swellings in the related zones that may feel like peas under the skin. These can also appear in the muscles, where they form spots of abnormal hardening. These used to be treated with painfully hard massages, but it turned out that gentle treatment here is just as efficient as a hard massage, especially when it is supplemented with the use of crystal wands and essential oils. This reflexology system may provide relief for many back problems, but since there is no "royal road" to healing lower-back pain, any reflexology treatment should be supported by physiotherapy, reasonable medication, and practices such as t'ai chi, qigong, yoga, or other exercises of inner awareness.

THE FOREARMS AND LOWER LEGS

Amazingly, even distant extremities like the forearms and lower legs contain reflexology systems. These zones were discovered in 1989 by Rudolf Siener, a German natural therapist who called these systems NPSO, for *Neue Punktuelle Schmerz- und Organtherapie* (in English, New Selective Pain and Organ Therapy). Acupuncture needles, electrical stimuli, and lasers are the main ways of treating these areas. These therapies have been shown to be effective in treating problems of the organs as well as for pain in the vertebral column.

Similarly, gentle massage of the front of the lower limbs has helped many people with different complaints—for example, constipation—which can be treated very effectively by massaging the relevant zones. These massages may be complemented with the use of diluted essential oil or with crystal wands.

In treatments performed by laypeople only very gentle touches should be used behind the knees above the calves for treatment of headaches. The rest of the calves should be excluded from massages—massage of this area could cause thrombosis. This risk doesn't apply to massage on the front side of the lower leg.

While the calves should not be massaged, they can be treated energetically with light touches. The individual performing the application should focus his or her mind on the energy in the hands. The hands will intuitively be attracted to those zones in need. Once the spot has been located it may feel as if the hand has been glued to it. A gentle touch without any movement on these spots balances the energy. Sometimes it takes only seconds; other times a zone requires up to two or three minutes to feel relief. A sure indication of success is a deep breath from the client, often accompanied by a sigh. At that point it's like the hand is released from that zone or point. This application can be used for tensions in the lower back, stiff neck, and headaches. For the latter ailment we may apply this technique quite successfully in the hollow of the knees.

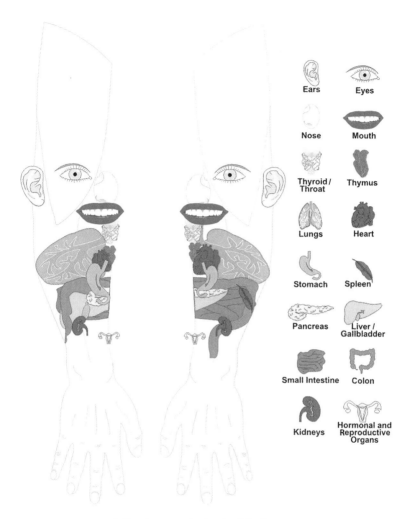

Ears   Eyes

Nose   Mouth

Thyroid /   Thymus
Throat

Lungs   Heart

Stomach   Spleen

Pancreas   Liver /
Gallbladder

Small Intestine   Colon

Kidneys   Hormonal and
Reproductive
Organs

Reflexology on the back of the forearm

The inside of the forearms can also be used to alleviate pain in all areas of the spine—lumbago, sciatica, cervical problems, and the consequences of whiplash injuries can be successfully treated if gently massaged. As a special application we can gently touch the inside of the elbow for alleviating headache. The back side of the forearm containing the organs is unfortunately not very convincing for organ treatments, but here massages have a good influence on disturbances

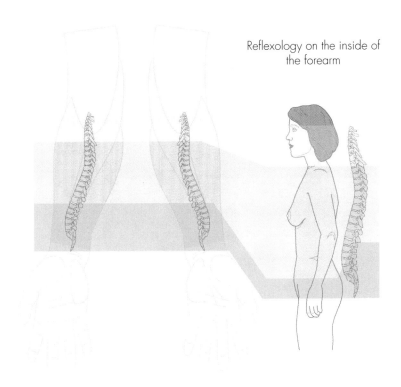

Reflexology on the inside of
the forearm

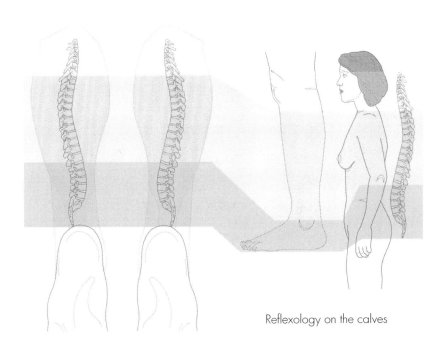

Reflexology on the calves

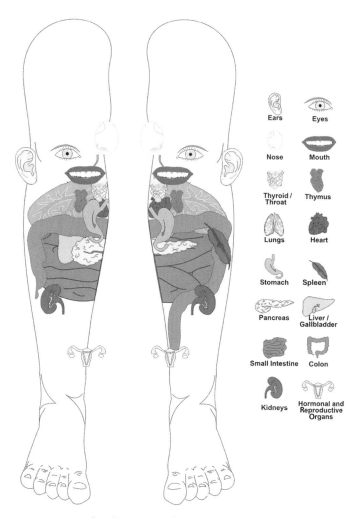

Ears

Eyes

Nose

Mouth

Thyroid /
Throat

Thymus

Lungs

Heart

Stomach

Spleen

Pancreas

Liver /
Gallbladder

Small Intestine

Colon

Kidneys

Hormonal and
Reproductive
Organs

Reflexology on the front of the lower leg

connected with the autonomous nervous system, such as nausea, hiccups, dizziness, light and sound sensitivity, and auras.

THE HANDS

Reflexology is commonly associated with the feet, while the possibilities of the hands are often overlooked. This is completely unjustified since hand reflexology is just as effective as foot reflexology. The hands, both on the palm and the back of the hand, serve physical as well as mental aspects. For physical symptoms, especially pain and functional complaints, hand reflexology can be quite effective. Hand massages are also an excellent self-treatment modality for enhancing well-being.

In addition to the physical aspects of hand reflexology there is also a psychospiritual dimension to this form of massage, as we may use the mudras (hand and finger positions that guide energy for overall health) to improve thinking. Sometimes certain signs that appear on the hands can be a warning that one's lifestyle is due to undergo some changes. These signs include red spots or an eczema that stays despite all kinds of treatments. The meaning behind these signs lies in our basic psychospiritual settings, where these are early warnings of a need to change one's attitude toward life or risk the physical consequences.

The hands need special "handling." For physical issues a series of reflexology massages are appropriate. Such a series of treatments promotes pain relief and stimulates an increased excretion of metabolic wastes. Examples are improvements of pain in the shoulder, an activation of the digestion, or better blood-pressure regulation. Medical professionals may apply acupuncture needles in the appropriate zones on the dorsal side of the hands; from this kind of treatment we can expect good effects on the movement apparatus and the metabolism.

In the mental or spiritual field visualizations like the balloon visualization described in part 4 can be used in conjunction with reflexology massage of both sides of the hands. This provides a gateway to the inner world, which paves the way for finding solutions when we feel stuck or answers to questions that concern us. Thus hand reflexology represents a holistic avenue for healing both physically and energetically in the whole person, body, mind, and spirit.

On the two hands one finds a microcosm of the whole human being in its three-dimensional structure. Only the feet are missing here.

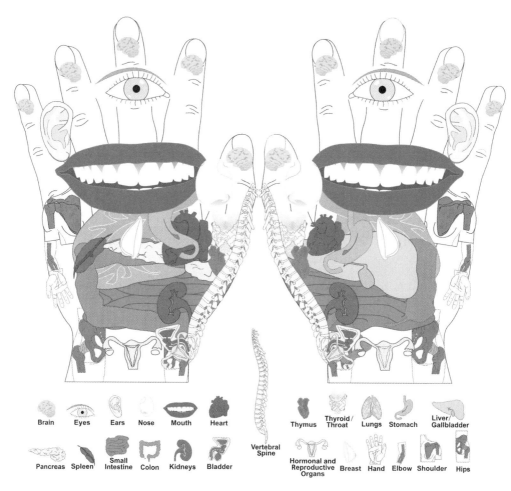

Reflexology on the back of the hand

There are three basic rules for reflexology on the hands: the left-right rule, the front-rear rule, and the top-bottom rule.

According to the left-right rule, the left side of the body is represented on the left hand, and disturbances in the right side appear on the right hand. Thus the left hip appears on the reflexology zones of the left hand and the right eye on the right hand. This also applies to the internal organs, where the appendix is to be found on the right hand, and the spleen is located in the reflexology zones on the left hand. For the spine we just need to put the two thumbs together. At

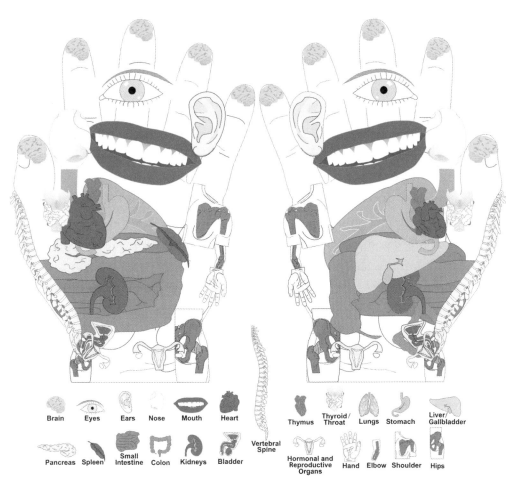

Reflexology on the palm of the hand

the meeting line the left half of the spine is on the left hand and the right half on the right hand.

As for the front-rear rule, we divide the body (with relaxed, hanging arms) into the front and the back. Attached to the front is the upper side of the hand, and to the back is the palm of the hands. Similarly, the nose and the belly are on the upper side of the hands, and the spine and the buttocks are located on the palm of the hands. The inner organs are on both sides of the hands.

For the top-bottom rule we divide the body into three areas: head with neck, chest, and pelvis with hips. As the fingers correspond to the head and neck the tops of the fingers correspond to the brain, and the sense organs have their zones. Below the end joint of the thumb, in the direction of the wrists, is the cervical spine zone. At the base joints of the fingers there is on the side of the thumb the transition between the cervical spine and the thoracic spine (between the red and the green area in the figure below), and on the lateral side of the hands the shoulder joints are found. One floor farther down (corresponding to the green area of the spine as shown in the figure below), toward the wrists, the zones on top of the metacarpals host the inner organs—the heart, lungs, stomach, gallbladder, liver, and pancreas. One floor farther down from this, at the carpal joints, the reflexology zones contain the lumbar spine, colon, small intestine, and the belly (the blue area of the spine). Finally, at the wrist is the sacrum (the orange area of the spine) along with the reproductive organs, the bladder, and the hip.

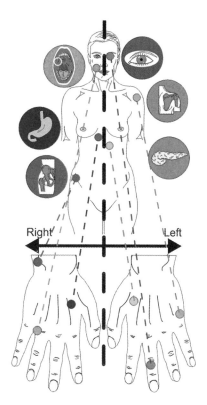

Reflexology system on the hand:
the left-right rule

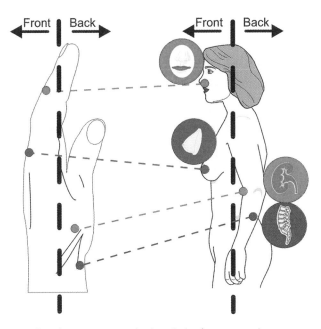

Reflexology system on the hand: the front-rear rule

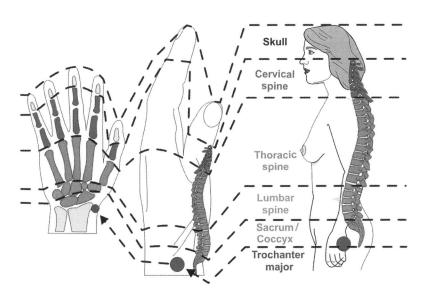

Reflexology system on the hand: the top-bottom rule

THE FINGERNAILS

This reflexology system, which has its origins in traditional Chinese medicine and ayurveda, seems quite unusual in that the information is mostly hidden under the fingernails and is not readily apparent upon cursory examination. American acupuncturist Gary Liscum, author, along with his wife, translator Zong Xiao-fan of *Chinese Medical Palmistry: Your Health in Your Hand,* points out that studies have shown that the microcirculation in the nail fold is very sensitive to changes in the entire organism. In the 1980s Liscum and Zong systematized their knowledge of Chinese medical diagnosis through the hands in a very clear way. The right side of the body is on the fingernails of the right hand, and the left side of the body on the left hand. In a top-down system the head with the brain has its representations under the thumbnails, with the left hemisphere on the left thumb and the right hemisphere on the right thumb, while the feet are under the fingernails of the little fingers, again with the left foot corresponding to the left little finger and the right foot to the right little finger. The remaining body zones are arranged proportionally under the other fingernails, as shown in the facing illustration.

This reflexology system is actually very simple and gives accurate diagnostic indications of disturbances in the body. After a slight pressure of about five seconds is applied to the nail the signs appear under the area where the nail is connected to the nail bed and remain visible for a few moments (naturally the fingernails should not be painted to use this test). A zone under the nail that remains whitish indicates a diminishing of energy or a chronic state in the associated organ. The opposite, circumscribed red spots appearing under the nail, shows an energetic overload with a tendency toward inflammation.

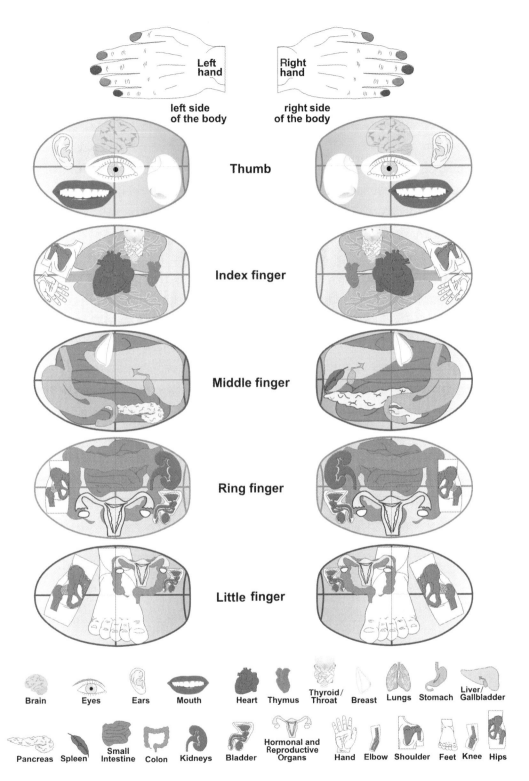

Reflexology of the fingernails

THE FEET

Our feet carry us through life, sometimes elatedly, sometimes reluctantly, sometimes angrily. Whatever way we choose to walk the feet are involved, so reflexology of the feet tells us how we are connected to the earth, especially as influenced by the metabolism. Accordingly we must always look at the signs on the feet from different perspectives—from the physical/metabolic aspect as well as from the mental/emotional aspect.

For example, let's consider athlete's foot as a common foot problem. This indicates a weakness of the immune system. Athlete's foot is not an insidious fungus that attacks us unawares; otherwise all people who use a swimming pool would have foot fungus. The areas where athlete's foot most frequently occurs are in the reflexology zones of the defense systems of the mouth and throat. Consequently athlete's foot is frequently accompanied by problems with the teeth or tonsils. In terms of mental/emotional matters it indicates that we have neglected our mental/emotional defenses and have opened the door to foreign colonization—outside thoughts and ideas are taking up too much space in our life.

With the first touch of a reflexology foot massage we can completely tune in to the other person. In a therapeutic setting reflexology massage of a client's feet opens new portals of healing. Massaging the feet of friends or partners is a powerful relaxation technique that promotes mutual understanding and fosters closeness. It is this range of possibilities that makes this system a special tool for health and well-being. There have been many studies from all over the world on the efficacy of reflexology foot massage:

- A 2009 University of Ulster study on the use of foot reflexology for the treatment of pain in people with multiple sclerosis showed "clinically significant improvements for MS symptoms."

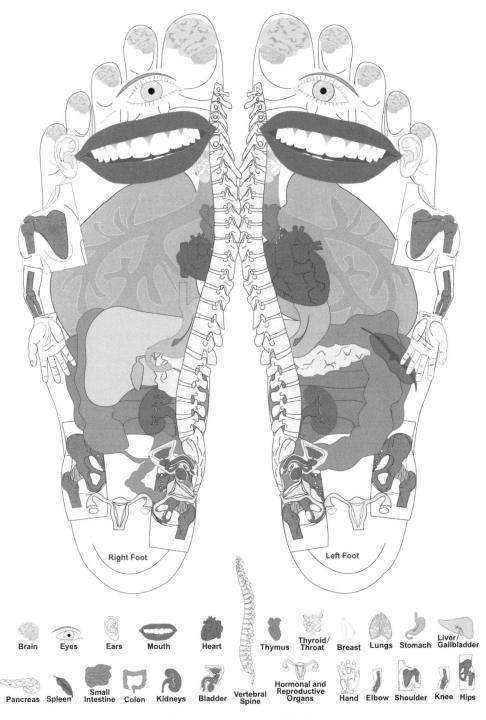

Reflexology on the soles of the feet

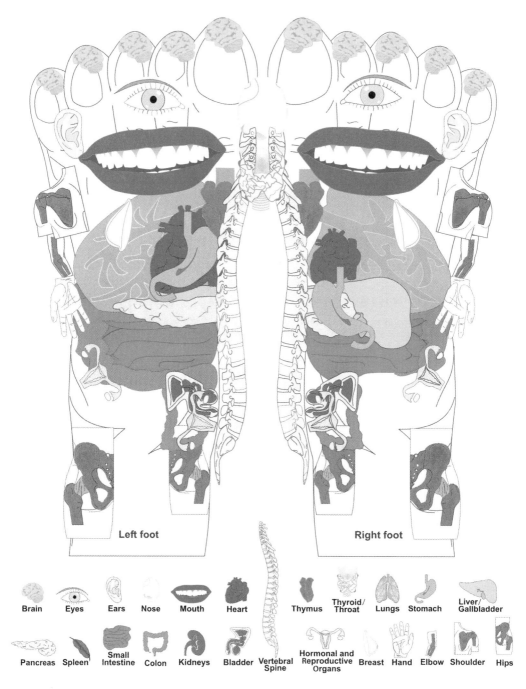

Left foot **Right foot**

Brain Eyes Ears Nose Mouth Heart Thymus Thyroid/Throat Lungs Stomach Liver/Gallbladder

Pancreas Spleen Small Intestine Colon Kidneys Bladder Vertebral Spine Hormonal and Reproductive Organs Breast Hand Elbow Shoulder Hips

Reflexology on the tops of the feet

- Kevin and Barbara Kunz, international authorities on the subject of reflexology, found significant improvements through foot reflexology after postoperative surgical care. Patients experienced an easing of pain, better sleep, less medication, and generally earlier discharge from the hospital (with a corresponding reduction of hospitalization costs). Through their organization, the Reflexology Research Project, they found overall improvements in the health and well-being of people diagnosed with cancer, phantom-limb syndrome, pregnancy, PTSD, and numerous other conditions, as documented at their website, www.reflexology-research.com.

- Through the use of functional magnetic resonance imaging (fMRI) technology scientists at the University of Hong Kong demonstrated that there is a correlation between areas in the brain responsible for movement and certain reflexology zones on the feet. This supports the use of reflexology to stimulate movement in people who have suffered a stroke.

These studies represent just the tip of the iceberg. Reflexology of the feet is effective at all levels of our being, including the human energy field. An example of the latter is the Metamorphic Technique pioneered in the late 1970s by Gaston Saint-Pierre, founder of the London-based Metamorphic Association, whose work was influenced by the prenatal therapy work of Robert Saint-John, a British naturopath and reflexologist. The premise of this healing technique is that during the nine months preceding birth all our physical, mental, emotional, and behavioral structures are laid down. Working on the spinal reflexes of the feet, hands, and head refocuses on this formative period, thus allowing healing to take place. This massage of the feet on the reflexology zones of the spine involves lightly stroking points that aim at the time of gestation. If a mother has stress or a bad experience during pregnancy the child may have certain problems later in approaching life, and we may find a disturbance in the associated reflexology zone.

In a meditative way we gently touch the zones, which feel energetically different. Using our intuition we remain fully attentive to that zone until there is a change in the energy quality. The results bring better connection to a person's purpose in life and an inner strength, a "coming home to the self."

All reflexology zones follow like a map of the human body on the feet, following the left-right rule that says that the left half of the body corresponds to the left foot and the right half of the body to the right foot, as shown on the facing page.

This is exactly the distribution of the reflexology zones. The imaginary line where the two feet meet when standing side-by-side represent the left and the right half of the spine. The sternum, the nose, and the abdominal muscles are in their halves of the body, and the same principle applies to the arrangement of the internal organs. From the center line and over each of the toes five vertical zones extend upward through the body. The big toe zone corresponds to the spinal column and goes up along the spine on the left and right sides, about two fingers' width from the vertebrae. Along this zone we also have the nose, the incisors, the esophagus, the aortic arch at the heart, the bladder, and the middle sections of the back muscles.

The next zone, to the left and right of the big toes, includes the middle corners of the eyes, the canines, the joints between the collarbones and the sternum, the gallbladder (right foot), and the lateral muscles of the back.

The next zone, more to the middle of the feet and corresponding to the middle toes, represents the eyeballs, the angles of the mouth, the middle of the collarbones, the breasts, and the ovaries.

One zone farther out along the extensions of both ring toes we have the cheek teeth, the joints between the collarbones and the shoulders, the lateral margin of the thoracic crest, the spleen (left foot), the ascending (right foot) and descending (left foot) colon, and the hip joints.

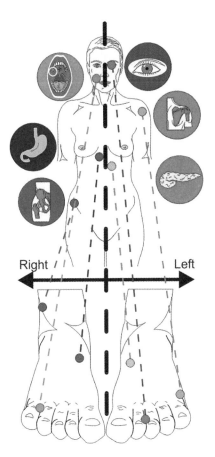

Foot reflexology—the left-right rule

Right   Left

In the last, the fifth, zone governing the little toes we find the ears, the jaw joints, the shoulder joints, the arms with the elbows and hands, and the trochanter major on the upper thighs. There are no internal organs in the little-toe zone as this corresponds mostly to the lateral parts of the body.

Now let's see how the front-back rule works in foot reflexology.

In the diagram on page 80 we see that the top of the two feet represents the front of the body and the soles the back of the body. Thus the nose, mouth, breastbone, breasts, navel, and abdominal muscles are found on the upper side of the feet, while the soles of the feet contain the zones of the back, the back muscles, and the buttocks. This also applies to the internal organs. While the lungs fill the entire chest and

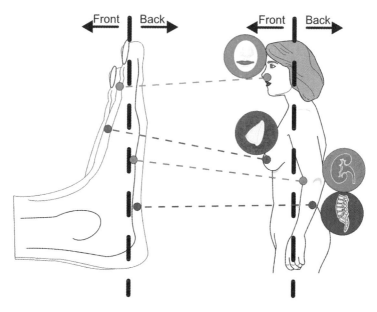

Foot reflexology—the front-back rule

thus are found on both the soles and on the instep, the gallbladder (right foot), thymus, breasts, and the urinary system are on the upper side of the feet, and the kidneys, spleen, and rectum are found on the soles.

Now let's consider the top-bottom rule as indicated by the floors delineated by the vertebral segments as shown on the facing page.

Here again a clear system is evident when we follow the floors from top to bottom. The first section starts at the head joints, at the transition between the first cervical vertebra and the skull, over the ears, to the front of the face over the eyebrows. This is the line formed by the upper edge of eyeglasses; on the feet this line corresponds exactly to the bottom end joints of the toes. In this zone where the spinal cord exits from the brain we find the vital switching points of the autonomic nervous system and the nerve cores of the cerebral nerves. These reflexology zones are in the flexion fold of the end joints of the big toes. In the tips of the toes and under the

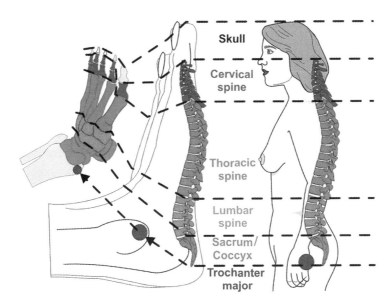

Foot reflexology—the top-bottom rule

toenails we find the zones of the brain. Accordingly the zones of the front of the brain and those of the forehead, including the frontal sinuses, are under the toenails, and the zones of the posterior brain are in the tips of the toes.

The next section goes through the joints between the toes and the metatarsals. This corresponds to the area between the seventh cervical vertebra and the first thoracic vertebra. Taking a closer look at this section, above this line are all the organs of the head, including the eyes, ears, nose, mouth, teeth, lymph drainage areas, thyroid, and cervical spine.

The next section passes through the joints between the metatarsals and the anterior tarsal bones. Transposed onto the body, this line begins between the twelfth thoracic vertebra and the first lumbar vertebra, then follows via the lower ribs on the left and right, and eventually connects in front in the line between the end of the bottommost rib pairs, known as the "floating ribs," halfway through the thoracic tip and the navel. This line corresponds to the diaphragm, and the section above it mainly includes the thoracic spine, the lungs and bronchi, and the heart.

Note that because the digestive organs (including the liver, gallbladder, pancreas, spleen, stomach, and intestines) move up and down through this line through the process of inhalation and exhalation, in foot reflexology they are located on a wide corridor above and below this line. However they can be precisely identified in foot reflexology as well as in other reflexology systems. For this we need the testing procedures described in part 3. The exact location of these organs on the feet demonstrates the limits of reflexology zone maps: precise as they may be, real precision can only be obtained by testing. Thus even the most accurate maps of reflexology only provide an approximation of the location of the organs.

The next line runs through the articular line between the anterior and the proximal tarsal bones. On the body this corresponds to a line that connects two transverse fingers below the navel at the front, following at the sides the upper edge of the pelvic scoops and going through the transition between the fifth lumbar vertebra and the sacrum. The section above this line contains, in addition to the lumbar spine, the kidneys and adrenal glands as well as the small intestine and the colon.

The last line passes through the upper ankle joints and corresponds to the pelvic floor in the body. In the section above this line are the sacrum, with the coccyx, the bladder, the sacroiliac joints, the vagina and the penis, the uterus and the prostate, and the rectum.

In addition to these lines demarcating the map of the body on the feet there are other significant points that show important functions. These include the outer and inner ankles as well as an imaginary ring around both lower limbs, about four transverse fingers above the ankles. The external nodules correspond to the left and right major trochanter. These bone mounds are anchoring points for the hip muscles that allow us to move on two legs.

These reflexology zones should always be included in the treatment of hip problems. The two inner ankle nodules are associated

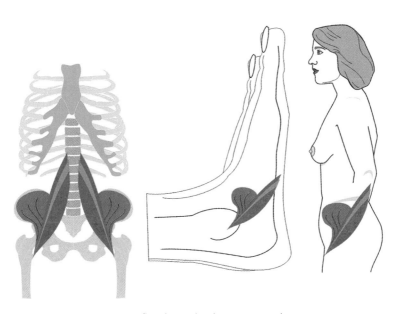

Foot reflexology: the iliopsoas muscle

with the left and right trochanter minor in foot reflexology. These bone mounds are the fixation points of the left and right iliopsoas muscles, which lift the thighs for walking or climbing stairs. Another important role comes from their basic function for energy production as they span the *hara* (or *dantien*), the energetic center of the body. At the same time, once both muscles of the iliopsoas are activated, they ensure in both sexes the advancing of the pelvis in sexual intercourse. Therefore, in case of chronic tension of these muscles, the joy of life will be impaired. Experience has shown that both the energy center and the sexual center can be enhanced by including these reflexology zones in foot massage.

3

. . . . . .

Diagnosis

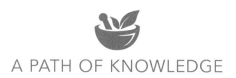

A PATH OF KNOWLEDGE

Before embarking on a course of treatment we must discover the obvious as well as the hidden sources of an ailment, so we must carefully examine the person we are treating. It is essential that we do so with an open mind and not bring our assumptions to the diagnosis; otherwise we will most likely find what we are looking for and overlook other crucial aspects that could help restore the person to health. The attitude that we bring to diagnosing should be one of openness, compassion, and mindfulness. In this way we will obtain all the information we need for effective treatment.

We begin our examinations in reflexology by using visual and tactile findings; in addition we use the elevator technique to determine the source of a condition as well as other testing procedures that are described here. All our findings should be verified by examining the same issue in a second or even a third reflexology system. Reflexology does not make medical diagnostics dispensable, but reflexology findings do provide an initial, fast orientation to the underlying problem; if the situation deems it, however, use conventional medicine's diagnostic technology as well.

The beginning of a session, when a diagnosis is made, often decides the course of treatment; this is a challenge for beginners as well as for experienced professionals. Your findings will point to where to focus your attention, leading the way to effective and successful treatment.

LOOKING AT THE SKIN

As simple as this may seem, visual inspection becomes multifaceted when one considers the different concepts involved: *seeing, viewing, scrutinizing,* and *observing,* to name a few ways we use our visual sense.

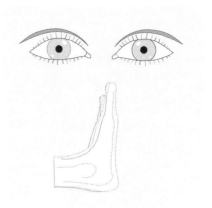

Looking and beholding, the two
modes of examination in reflexology

In reflexology two ways of inspecting are useful: to *look at* and *to behold*.

When we look at a reflexology area the focus is on color and structural changes on the skin as a possible contrast to the general appearance of healthy skin. A different approach is beholding, as this is a kind of open-minded contemplation. Many signs do not make sense at first glance, and yet they have an underlying meaning. Insight into the meaning can only be gained by regarding beyond the mind's usual way of thinking—by beholding. Start out by looking at a reflexology zone, allowing the gaze to rest at some point or structural formation. Then ruminate in a compassionate way. When we look respectfully, with the heart as well as the eyes, we get a deeper level of information. Then we can assign to our mind the task of sorting through our impressions. The basis of this technique lies in the processing mode of the brain. As pointed out already, the intuitive right half of the brain works much faster than the left hemisphere, the analytical half of the brain, so in beholding we are using a combination of both faculties.

So begin with the first level of visual assessment, looking at the skin. Some of the typical signs useful in reflexology display the following characteristics:

- **Pale zones:** Pale, cool skin areas may be considered an expression of a lack of energy, which applies to the corresponding organ in that zone. This may be the result of exhaustion or an indicator of a chronic condition.

- **Skin inclusions:** These include all types of cutaneous (skin) cysts such as epidermal inclusion cysts, the result of the implantation of epidermal elements in the dermis, as well as such harmless presentations as deposits of fat or tallow under the skin. Sometimes the body uses the skin as a disposal platform where we get rid of substances we cannot otherwise eliminate. In particular, residues of heavy metals or pesticides may find their way out of the body in this way. These and even more serious inclusions should be medically clarified. Fatty or tallow compounds may be regarded as metabolic dumping sites. These we find not only under the skin; calcareous deposits (i.e., stones) in the gallbladder or kidneys belong to this same category. The body organizes these deposits when the metabolic function is reduced—that is, the "garbage collection" system is not working properly.

- **Calluses:** Areas of calloused skin usually reveal that the corresponding muscle systems are chronically tense, which means a reduction of energy and blood supply. On the feet and hands such calluses mostly develop in areas associated with the shoulder and hip muscles. Of course should you have worked a weekend in the garden with a hoe and shovel, the calluses on your hands are due to mechanical causes and are not reflexology signs.

- **Pimples:** Pimples are signs that the body is trying to squeeze something out through the skin, something we absolutely need to get rid of. This way the body discharges metabolic wastes, substances the metabolism can no longer eliminate through normal channels.

- **Red zones:** Red, hot, or inflamed areas on the skin show a process of irritation or even inflammation in the related organ. In the background we will often find an overreaction or a defensive fight under way in the immune system.

- **Warts:** Deposits in the form of warts are mental formations making a physical appearance. It is always amazing how easily warts disappear without a trace when thoughts are changed or the mind is cleared. Sometimes it is necessary to support this process with ritual. Our ancestors' methods for removing warts speak volumes as to the mental source of the problem: magic twine, spider's legs, or certain conjuring formulas are some of the many methods that were used in the past to treat warts—proof enough that warts are formations that literally come from the mind.

TACTILE ASSESSMENT

After an initial visual inspection we next scan the reflexology system with our hands for conspicuous tactile signs. This is to determine if there is any tissue tension or signs in the subcutaneous tissue. The muscles play only a negligible role in this palpation. The most important tactile findings are swellings and skin condensing. If a zone is swollen it will feel like a fluid-filled pillow under the skin. Swellings have the meaning of too much energy in the zone and the associated

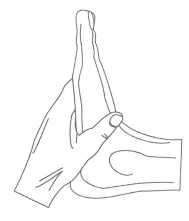

Tactile assessment

organ. If in palpating we feel compressed skin that could also appear as nodules or a hardening in the skin, this indicates a state of low energy.

The technique for tactile assessment in reflexology involves circling with a finger five or six times on the spot with gentle pressure and then moving to the next spot—a bit like traveling on the skin from one point to the next. Since the focus of this skin palpation is the connective tissue under the skin, we should not glide on the surface of the skin and should use only a small amount of oil. At conspicuous points we may examine the zone with a deeper touch. As with all the other examination techniques, neither circling nor palpation should be painful.

The beginning of that finger journey should be, if possible, along the reflexology zone of the spine. This can be performed from the zone of the head, working toward the pelvis, or the other way around, from the pelvis to the head. The crucial element is to go all the way up or down the spine, not skipping any floors. This is the basis of the elevator technique, a testing method I will describe below, in the section on energetic testing methods. After this, scan the reflexology system with a circling palpation in vertical tracks, or just use your intuition, allowing your hands to probe without thinking, using open-minded, compassionate beholding. The HeartMath Institute has found that we are interconnected through the electromagnetic fields of the heart. This means that when listening to our heart and not to our mind we can act on our inner navigation device and thus be led to the zones that are the most important to be treated.

ENERGETIC TESTING METHODS

Before starting a treatment find the point or zone that will yield long-lasting effects. Certain tests based on kinesiology have proved to be most effective for this purpose, because they directly engage the body's wisdom. Muscle testing is the simplest and most accurate way to get

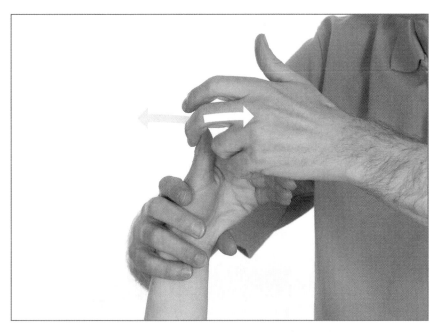

Muscle testing is based on the principles of kinesiology.

answers. This can be done with the thumb or the big toe or with a pendulum; if you are familiar with pulse testing that is a suitable alternative.

Because kinesiology uses contact with a person's subconscious it is extremely important that we mentally clear ourselves before starting the test and not expect any particular results by mentally imagining them. Otherwise we will obtain the answer we want and not that required by the person being treated. In addition we must always ask permission before any kind of muscle test to see whether we are permitted to ask this type of question. And after every test result we owe the subconscious mind of the person being tested a silent *thank you* for its willingness to communicate. Asking these questions of a person's deep inner psyche should never be taken for granted; it is only through respect and gratitude for this process that we obtain a good connection, with clear answers. As well, in both testing and treatment we obtain the best results if we breathe along with the client. During

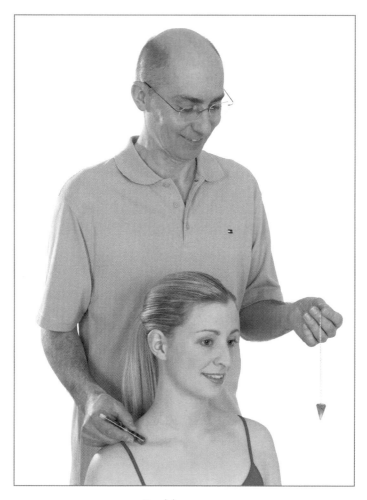

Pendulum testing

testing always pay attention to your breathing and that of the person you are treating.

Kinesiology has a long and well-documented tradition, and there is a wealth of literature to refer to, so I will not go into great detail here on its underlying principles and instead will focus on three user-friendly *yes/no* questions by which you can get good results regardless of the method you use. Note that muscle testing should *never* be used for anything other than to respond to a simple *yes* or *no* question.

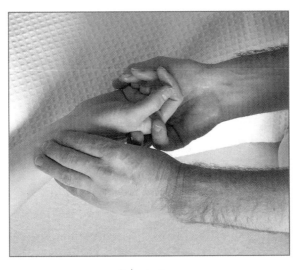

Pulse testing

The following instructions apply to any method of muscle testing, whether using the thumb or big toe, or using a pendulum (or even a dowsing rod), because the agreement/rejection response always encompasses the whole person—body, mind, and spirit. That said, we have found that we obtain the clearest signals using the thumb or the big toe to test.

Calibrating Yes and No

Before beginning the test determine the indicators for *yes* and *no*. This is called *calibration,* and it entails asking the client about positive and negative experiences to determine a *yes* and *no* response when muscle testing. When testing it is very important not to ask about people or events, as doing so may evoke annoyance, denial, or other strong emotions, which will in turn cause defensive mechanisms to mobilize and elicit a *yes* in a *no* situation, and vice versa.

So that the person you are treating will know what you are looking for in terms of resistance, push with a little bit of pressure against her thumbnail (or big toenail) while asking her to lightly resist the pressure. Then let go. This is not some kind of measure of strength, so only apply a little pressure. More is not necessary.

After your internal breath attunement to your client, begin by asking her for a clear, agreeing *yes*. To do this you might want to employ a visualization: ask her to imagine that she is sitting at a table and that her favorite dish is placed, piping hot, in front of her. Allow a few moments for the image to emerge, and when you see that the look on her face indicates that she is enjoying the dish, or if you perceive a nod, then silently say, *please test now,* and press lightly for one to three seconds (no longer) against the thumb or the big toe. You will then notice that the thumb or big toe of the client remains stable in its joint and holds steady against the pressure. Then give a silent thanks and let go. In this manner you have obtained the *yes* signal via a strong muscle response.

Then ask your client for a clear, rejecting *no*. As a suggesion to elicit this response you could ask her to imagine something she really does not like at all, that she finds distasteful, or even ask her to imag-

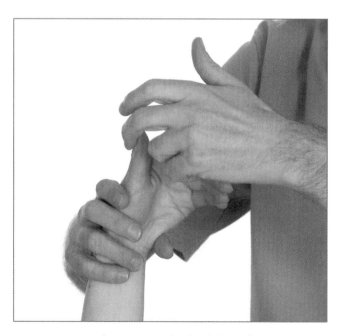

Test indicating *yes*—the thumb holds firm

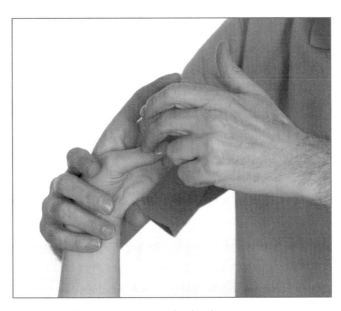

Test indicating *no*—the thumb gives way

ine a situation in which she felt weak. Look for the body's expression, and then say, *please test now* and press briefly for one to three seconds against the thumb or big toe. You will notice that the thumb or big toe of the person bends at the joint. Thus you have obtained a *no* via a weak muscle response.

You now have clarified the *yes* and *no* signals with the person's subconscious and are ready to proceed to test for the specific treatment to be used. But first you must ask permission to continue. Ask, "Is it acceptable for us to test?" Silently saying, *please test now,* apply light pressure on the thumb or the big toe. A strong muscle indicates permission to continue with testing. If a *no* comes up, we have to respect it and choose a different way to proceed.

Using the Elevator Technique

When William Fitzgerald delineated the reflexology system found on the feet more than a hundred years ago he found that it corresponds to the anatomical layout of the body. At about the same time the structure of the nervous system was described for the first time. With these two breakthroughs it became apparent that all organs and body structures are connected to the electrical impulse currents in the spinal column via the associated floors, the horizontal levels defined by the vertebral segments. This can be compared to an elevator in a high-rise building. Each floor in the building is serviced by the elevator. Similarly the body operates based on the stream of information that runs through the spinal cord; specifically through each floor, each of which provides information related to certain organs, movement structures, and even associated mental/emotional patterns. Reflexology uses this information for examination and treatment.

In using this elevator technique the reflexology zones of the spinal column are checked for disturbances. If an active zone or point (i.e., a disturbance) is identified it refers not only to the spinal column itself but also to the entire floor ruled by that segment. This means that at the point of disturbance we will explore the organs and body structures supplied by that segment. If no disturbance is found in the floor's organs and body structures we can assume that the disturbance in the segment relates to the spine itself.

To return to the elevator metaphor: We can compare this technique to someone who is troubleshooting in a high-rise building in which the top twenty-nine floors serviced by the elevator are called *cervical,* the next seven are called *thoracic,* the next twelve after that are called *lumbar,* the next five are called *sacral,* and the final four, including the ground floor, are called *coccyx.* The elevator we take is equipped with a warning light. In our body the elevator is the spinal column, the warning light is the disturbance found in the vertebral floor, and the troubleshooting is the test to determine which organ system, movement structure, or spinal segment is disturbed.

As we ascend the elevator the spine will register an alarm at any floor where something is wrong. This disruption is called the *leader.* This is the reflex zone that indicates the overall theme, the one that can resolve the issue, the crux of the matter. There we stop, open the

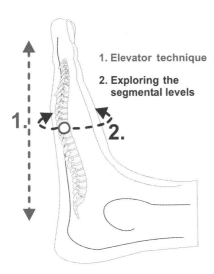

1. **Elevator technique**

2. **Exploring the segmental levels**

Elevator technique on the foot

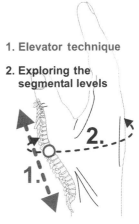

1. **Elevator technique**

2. **Exploring the segmental levels**

Elevator technique on the hand

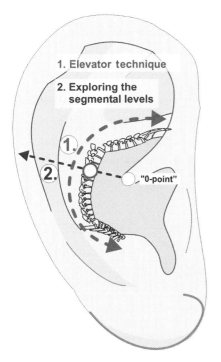

1. **Elevator technique**

2. **Exploring the segmental levels**

"0-point"

Elevator technique on the ear

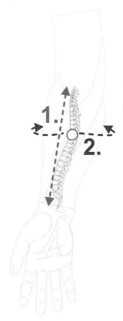

1. **Elevator technique**

2. **Exploring the segmental levels**

Elevator technique on the elbow

door of the elevator, and proceed to look around that level for the nature of the disturbance. For this exploration within this level we follow a broad corridor. The organs have their connections to the spine via the autonomic nervous system. Where we encounter a dysfunctional organ the nervous-system impulses converge to sound an alarm in the corresponding reflexology zone. Usually as soon as that reflex zone is unblocked everything within that zone unblocks in a cascading domino effect.

In using the elevator technique to explore the floors to determine what needs treatment, two testing methods that complement each other are employed: tactile assessment and muscle testing. In tactile assessment the reflexology zones of the spine are traversed in small circles, with attention to any irregularities in the subcutaneous tissue. This is followed by an exploration of the reflexology floors in the same way. Using the muscle test, ask the client to show a strong *yes,* then slowly trace along the reflexology zone of the spinal floor with a finger or a crystal wand. For this it doesn't matter whether we go from the occiput to the coccyx or the other direction, from the bottom up. Ask the client to maintain a *yes* for the entire search up or down the elevator. At a troubled point—the leader—the signal changes to a *no.* At this point stop and allow the person to relax. Now ask the client to activate the *yes* again, then proceed to explore that floor. The disturbed organ or structure will reveal itself; the muscle of the thumb (or big toe) will get weak again, indicating a *no* signal. Again, note that all organs doing well will provide a *yes* response, and only disturbances will show up with a *no* response. So if you silently say the name of the organ or organs associated with a certain floor during your exploration and get a *no* response, you'll know that the organ is in a disturbed state.

The elegance of the elevator technique lies in its fast and precise accuracy. In the past only the pain reactions of a person were reliable indicators of a disturbance, and so determining which organ was involved was a matter of assumption or even speculation. The elevator technique combined with muscle testing provides us with clear answers through communication with the subconscious, which never lies.

Testing for Essential Oils and Crystals

When using essential oils and/or crystal wands in a treatment, muscle testing makes it clear which oil or crystal is best suited for the treatment. After detecting the reflexology zone that needs support, intuitively choose from four or five oils or crystals, based on whether you will need to activate a depleted energy condition or calm an overstimulated condition (to determine this, see part 4, page 107, "Activating or Calming?"). Now touch the relevant zone with the bottle of oil or the crystal, put it down, then test your client for *yes* or *no*. Another way you can test for crystals is to hold one in one hand while testing with the other hand. With essential oils you can swipe the scent under the client's nose, then test for *yes* or *no*. The *yes* response, indicated by a strong thumb or toe, will be best for the treatment.

Observing Minimal Clues

Nonverbal communication from the person we are treating offers a wealth of information that can be very useful in reflexology. Communications experts have long known that most communication occurs on the unconscious level. In 1970 anthropologist Ray Birdwhistell of the University of Pennsylvania published the results of his groundbreaking studies on nonverbal communication in his book *Kinesics and Context: Essays on Body Motion Communication*. Birdwhistell found that nonverbal communication prevails over verbal communication in almost every social interaction. These kinds of studies have been repeated over the years, with similar results every time. For example, in one of his studies it was found that in normal conversation about 38 percent of meaning is conveyed through tonality, through things such as voice timbre, accent, or talking speed; 55 percent of meaning occurs nonverbally, including facial expression, posture, breathing pattern, and gestures; and only 7 percent of meaning occurs through actual words. Therefore 93 percent of our communication—what I call *minimal clues*—occurs unconsciously.

As for facial expression, we know that most expressions are regulated by the neurotransmitter dopamine, which plays a major role in reward-motivated behavior. Once there is a release of this hormone the face gets the appearance of the person being in a good mood; if, on the other hand, dopamine is lacking, the face has the appearance of disappointment and unhappiness. All this occurs without our even being aware of it, but others around us receive these unconscious signals, oftentimes reacting to them unawares.

We can use these unconscious signals or minimal clues advantageously in reflexology. For example, when we calibrate for *yes* and *no* on a client using different scenarios, we may notice that with a wonderful *yes* the person's shoulders relax, there is deep, full breathing, and the facial expressions speak of approval. On the other hand, a disgusted *no* shows the opposite: the shoulders tense and lift up slightly, the eyes get

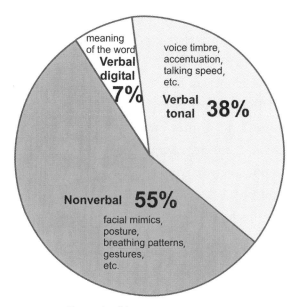

Channels of human communication
(Ray Birdwhistell, University of Pennsylvania)

narrow, the angles of the mouth sink, and breathing becomes shallower, from the chest instead of the belly.

To observe minimal clues we must shift from one-pointed focus to opening and broadening our vision. A proven technique consists of looking through the person to a point at some distance behind him or her. In this way of looking we can operate physiologically, in defocused vision, which allows us to register changes in a wider sense. For example, when observing minimal clues while using the elevator technique on the foot reflexology zones, we'll find that the breathing pattern remains in the *yes* mode, regular and relaxed, as we glide along the reflexology zone of the spine. When we hit a disturbance the breathing pattern switches over to a *no* signal—the breath becomes stagnant or even halting, or there is some noticeable change. Noticing these subtleties takes some experience, but once we attune to the minimal clues found in nonverbal communication it provides a wealth of information to support our work.

4
......
Techniques

PREPARING FOR PRACTICE

Reflexology can be used for basic health and well-being and to alleviate minor complaints as well as to treat certain chronic disease conditions. When using reflexology for health and well-being, supplementing with essential oils or crystals can enhance the experience and facilitate self-exploration, thereby deepening one's self-awareness. In therapeutic applications medical professionals can use acupuncture needles, lasers, or electrical stimulation on relevant reflexology points to improve disorders and disease conditions. Beyond these applications though, reflexology has an additional benefit: it helps a person regain her or his own innate healing powers and connect to their innermost being.

The most important tools in using reflexology are natural ones: our heart and our hands. The goal is to give impulses for health and well-being. This means that we must foster the image of a healthy, contented human being. If we orient ourselves in the wrong way, by doing battle, trying to fight an ailment, we will send out the wrong energetic impulses. And even if our intention is correct we are never in a position to *impose* health on another person. Health grows within each person—we can only give the impulses to the organism for achieving health. And even in that regard there are a few traps in reflexology that should be considered.

The first one, just mentioned, is the belief that we can heal others. The second trap is the assumption that the more we do, the more it will help. In all treatments it is neither the strength of the pressure applied nor the amount of time we apply it that is relevant. It is rather the intensity of the inner connection with what we do and the quality of communication with the other person that determines the success of a treatment. When this happens we will be guided through mutual understanding to focus on a reflexology point for the right amout of time, and we'll have perfect timing in our sessions every time.

A third trap for holistic practitioners paradoxically lies in having too much sympathy. Of course treatment without compassion is inhuman—cold and technical. Without compassion there is no inner connection, either with ourself or with the other person. But the other extreme, joining a client in his or her suffering, is equally ineffective, as we are caught in the helper syndrome, becoming helpless helpers. Thus it is only in an appreciation of the strength and the beautiful aspects of our clients that we can escape these traps. This is the attitude to bring to treatment, where health is nourished and can grow within the person who has entrusted him- or herself to us. This way, with every treatment our clients get healthier, and we foster our own health as well.

Another aspect in practicing reflexology of which we should be aware is the transfer of energies. Occasionally you will encounter clients who unconsciously tap in to your energy system, with the result being that you feel drained after a session. The person certainly didn't do this consciously or intentionally. But if they are exhausted or have gone through hard times, this tapping in to another's energy reserves can be an inner, unconscious survival strategy. Another way clients tap in to your energy is when there is a heavy disease involved, like cancer or multiple sclerosis. Experience has shown that these chronic illnesses produce a huge amount of energy—the energy of worry and fear—and people who suffer from these kind of conditions have to get rid of that excess energy. That is probably one reason why these people are better off if they get a pet, a dog or a cat. Animals can much more easily take on the surplus energy and ground it in the matrix of nature. But when we practitioners are exposed to these energies we have to deal with them. In the beginning of my work as a medical massage therapist I did not realize this. It was only later, with more experience working with subtle energy, that I figured this out. There are a number of techniques you can use as protection—one is to use a protective cocoon of light while working. However, as good as your technique is, it can sometimes reduce the contact with the other person and consequently the flow of information. Therefore my own personal solution is to connect myself to the main universal source of energy while working, allowing it to flow through me. Then it is insignificant whether a client taps in to my energy as they will only get their "fair share" from the universal source in which I am grounded.

A Simple Protection Technique

The following technique can be used before and after a treatment; it only takes three breaths to establish within oneself that stream of universal power that protects us.

1. The first breath (inhalation plus exhalation) is to connect yourself via your imaginary roots with the core of the earth.
2. With the second breath open yourself to the light of the universe, the source of energy.
3. With the third breath establish a beam of light running from the stars, through your body, to the center of the earth, with your body as a conductor of this universal energy.

In this way you can remain untouched by the energies of clients. In fact it allows you to be fully aware of any attempt to latch on to your personal energy—a realization that gives additional options for treatment strategies.

The following is an alternative protective technique, a visualization you can do before seeing a client that only takes a few moments and allows you to connect with the source of universal energy and, in so doing, offers protection.

———————— ⌒ ————————

Sit comfortably, or stand in a stable position, your feet planted firmly on the ground. Put your hands below the navel, resting on your *hara,* your energy center. With the first breath imagine your feet putting down roots. As you continue to breathe, let these roots spread ever deeper and deeper into the earth until they reach the earth's inner core of magma. Let your roots splash joyously in the magma and watch as all your stressful thoughts and emotions flow out to it. The earth, with her unimaginable power, can easily transform these influences. Splash around in the magma for two or three breaths. With the next breath open your imaginary sunroof at the crown of your head and turn your attention to the starry sky. One of the stars winks at you, and its light flows down through your sunroof, down through your spine, and down your roots into the magma at the center of the earth. On the last breath enjoy the whirlpool of light bubbles around your roots. You now exist as a beautiful, light-filled connection between the outer universe and the inner earth. You feel how wonderful it is to be a mediator, a conductor of primordial energy. With this solid anchor in the earth and a powerful stream of light energy from the cosmos, you can start the treatment.

———————— ⌒ ————————

ACTIVATING OR CALMING?

No matter which reflexology system you are using, a crucial determination at the outset is whether you are treating an energy-deficient state or an energy-excess state, and for this you must test. Use any of the testing methods described in this book: muscle testing with thumb or big toe, pendulum testing, pulse testing—all work well for this purpose. In the case of a deficiency of energy you must conduct energy to a point and its associated organ; in the case of an excess of energy you will need to disperse energy away from the point and its associated organ. Any disturbance is related to one or the other energetic state. Energy deficiencies are mostly due to chronic conditions or mentally burdening situations that have been going on for a long time. Energy excesses have to do with more exuberant processes, like inflammation or a sudden, intense emotional challenge.

As well, keep in mind that quick strokes with more intense pressure applied are activating. Slow, gentle strokes are balancing.

If you are using a crystal wand or essential oil in the reflexology massage, test to see which stones or oils are appropriate for either conducting energy toward or away from an area. Also see the overview tables beginning on pages 120 and 124.

THE IMPORTANCE OF CORRECT MASSAGE TECHNIQUE

Massage is one of the oldest healing modalities of humankind. In the truest sense of the word we touch another person and in so doing allow ourselves to be touched by the experience of the flow of energy between two people. Massage means soothing grasps, targeted attention, and the exchange of energy via direct physical contact. All this applies even more so in reflexology, since it uses all these aspects in a very differentiated, energetic way.

The beginning of a massage is about getting to know the other person. We want to gain a general impression of him or her, while the person on the receiving end needs to have a favorable impression about us as well. How do the hands feel? Do I like the touch, is it enjoyable to be touched by these hands? So the client's first contact with our hands is essential, as there is a flow of information coming from both sides. We should therefore get into this experience consciously. Start by holding the person's feet, back, or any other treatment area for three or four deep breaths before doing anything. This is when we synchronize our breath with the client's, modeling full, complete breathing that fosters connection and acceptance. On this basis health, well-being, and healing can arise.

Massaging means that we always feel and act at the same time. However this only happens when the work of our hands comes from

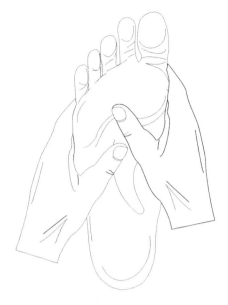

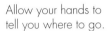
Allow your hands to
tell you where to go.

our hara, the energetic center located just below the navel. With our attention at the hara, our hands hardly have to work at all, as they become extensions of our consciousness. This is even more true in reflexology, where oftentimes we are led to the points or zones that the hands just seem to gravitate toward. Therefore the best way to massage is to start out by letting our hands mindfully follow our heart, which is how we can connect with the electromagnetic field of the person we are massaging.

Yin and Yang in Massage

After these first few moments of contact, continue stroking according to the principles of yin and yang. In traditional Chinese medicine yin is the front of the body, where the energy flows upward, and yang is the back, where energy has a downward direction. This means that the strokes on the front should go from the toes to the head, and the strokes on the back should go from the head to the toes. On the feet, for example, the yin strokes go upward from the heels over the upper side of the feet toward the toes, and the yang strokes run downward

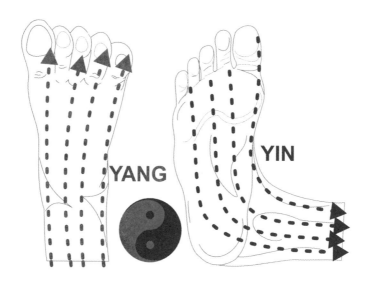

Yin and yang strokes in foot reflexology

in the opposite direction, over the soles. These yin and yang strokes balance the energies. In general our strokes should pull, and we must avoid any pushing.

We each have our own personal way of using our hands in massage. Big hands will massage differently than small hands, but again, it is not the force of our hands that decides the effectiveness of a massage. As long as we massage with mindfulness our hands will act as performing tools. Then the energies can flow, and the adequate amount of power will be available. We will get confirmation that our massage technique is right when the person who has entrusted him- or herself to our hands falls asleep or sighs contentedly.

In addition to the yin-yang direction of strokes, we should make our hands as soft as possible and mold them to the reflexology area that we treat. I have found that the trick is to consciously pay attention to the relaxation of the little fingers while massaging. Once they feel soft the hands can model around the skin and lie evenly on the surface. Then it is irrelevant whether we are working on the back of the feet, the neck, or the contours of the hands.

STROKES

In reflexology, the techniques we use to massage are circling on the spot, cat's stepping, pincer grasp, and the mobilization of joints. Let's look at each in detail.

Circling on the Spot

This massage technique can be both investigative and therapeutic, and depending on the intensity it will have a stimulating, neutral, or calming effect. Fast, vigorous circles will concentrate energy into a zone, whereas slow and soft circles are soothing and energy dispersing. For this technique, circle around one point, always remaining in contact with the skin, without sliding. If using a crystal wand follow the same procedure. After about five to seven circles move to the next point, overlapping with the previous massage circle as you go.

This technique can be used to feel the structures of the connective tissue under the skin. It can also be used as a means to spread relaxation into the surrounding tissue after the basic unblocking procedure (described in the next section) or to tone the tissue. Please carry out these circling movements very slowly, in time with the breathing rhythm of your client.

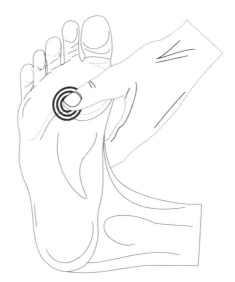

Circling on the spot

If you follow your intuition the direction of movement of these circles is generally unimportant. However if you should sense an inner resistance to a direction, or sense tension, or you notice an autonomic reaction in your client, simply change directions. An autonomic nervous–system reaction in reflexology massage might involve goose bumps, light perspiration, spontaneous need to urinate, increased flow of saliva, or dryness of the mouth, to name a few. All these spontaneous sensations indicate that the nervous system is having "digestive problems" with the incoming impulses.

Circle Direction

With circles there is always the question of whether to massage clockwise or counterclockwise. Which is activating and which is relaxing? Which is correct and which should be avoided? The answer lies in your own intuition, in following your hands. And if you are unsure or in doubt, there is an easy test: Circle a few times in one direction and then in the other direction while holding your thumb against the client's thumb and applying slight pressure. The direction of circling that yields good muscle strength is the correct direction. The direction where the thumb feels weak is wrong.

Cat's Steps

This is a soft, rhythmic massage technique that uses alternating soft thumb pressure in a kind of movement that we know from cats before they snuggle into a place they like. This technique is especially useful for addressing the reflexology zones of the autonomic nervous system, the intestines, and the chakras. It calms and balances the whole energy situation of the body and the mind.

Pincer Grasp

When working on the head zones and shoulder zones of the feet and the hands, this grip is very useful. These reflexology zones are taken

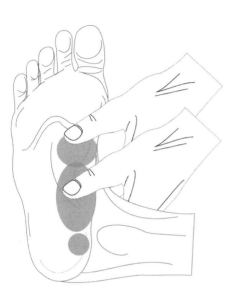

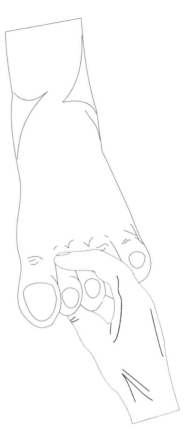

Cat's steps calms and
balances the energy of
the body and mind.

The pincer grasp is an effective
technique for influencing the
head and shoulders.

between the thumb and index finger. The zones are then massaged
with circular movements, with a pumping action or with soft pulling.
This technique allows us to directly influence the head and shoulders
via reflexology. In this way we can massage the teeth, the organs of the
senses, the lymphatic system, and the throat.

Mobilization of the Joints

When reflexology treatment is given with the heart and the hands
as it should, the client will often dive in to a state of deep relaxation

between being awake and asleep, like drifting away with the mind in outer space. Now at the end of a massage it is our task to guide the person smoothly back into reality, even if they like staying in this state. Holding one foot and then the other at the end of a treatment and gently moving all joints of the foot serves this purpose.

Start by holding the toes as a whole with one hand and the metatarsal bones of the forefoot with the other hand in a strong but gentle grip. Now, for about fifteen seconds, slowly move the hands in small movements against each other as you would move the pedals of a bicycle. Then repeat this procedure a little bit higher, between the forefoot and the anklebone (talus). The third grip is then between the anklebone and the heel bone.

There are receptors for our upright equilibrium in all the ligaments and joint capsules (the envelopes surrounding the synovial joints) of the feet. When walking over rough, uneven surfaces in everyday life these receptors are activated to become more attentive and alert.

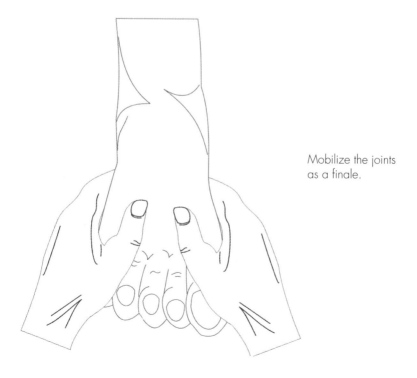

Mobilize the joints as a finale.

Gently mobilizing the joints of the feet conveys exactly these same messages to the brain. Slowly the person will open her eyes and return to her surroundings. Additionally, because this technique loosens the deep structures of the feet, by awakening her in this way she will leave the treatment feeling refreshed and joyful.

BASIC UNBLOCKING TECHNIQUE

One of the central techniques in reflexology is the basic unblocking technique. In life as in reflexology, sometimes the most effective things turn out to be the easiest things, and the basic unblocking technique is really easy. Once we find an unbalanced reflexology point, the leader (any point or zone that we've determined is disrupted, as described previously), we calmly press that point with one finger without any other movement, gradually increasing the pressure until we perceive a change in the person's breathing. It may be a small stopping of the breath, a change in the depth of the breath, a twitching, a hesitation, or a falter. Stay with exactly this amount of pressure for about ten to twenty seconds. Sometimes just a mere touch elicits this sensation, and other times we must apply more

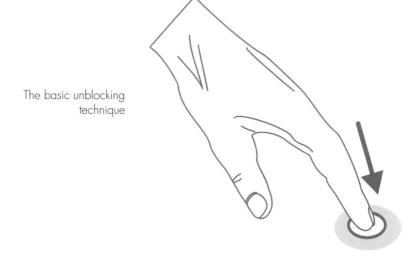

The basic unblocking technique

intense pressure; but in any case stay just below the pain threshold, until your finger sinks into the tissue and you observe the client breathing deeply again as the spot softens. Quite often this is accompanied by a sigh. This is a sign that you are in contact with the client's body awareness and that you have permission from those deeper levels of her being to proceed further. Basic unblocking is, so to speak, a conversation with the client's inner healing wisdom.

What do you do if the point does not release even after thirty seconds? This is a clear message that we should leave this reflexology zone, ease off on the area with some gentle strokes, and continue with another point. If that unbalanced point is along the spinal column we'll need to look for an organ in the relevant reflexology segment. On the other hand, if we find such a reflexology point that does not react according to expectations in the course of a general palpation or massage in a reflexology system, we should pay attention to the vertebral column and explore the associated segment of the spine. Sometimes it indicates that there is a more important issue that needs to be treated first. For that muscle testing is the best way to determine which issue needs to be addressed. After all, the body is always right, even if we sometimes don't believe it.

Balloon Visualization

Holistic practitioners know that body, mind, and spirit are not separate. This is in fact the premise of all forms of natural healing. The link between our physical, mental, and spiritual parts are to be found in the autonomic nervous system and in the communication that occurs between the cells. In practice we use imagery to address our inner wisdom, which controls our physical processes and influences cell communication. Therapeutic hypnosis and visualization have long been known to achieve incredible results in ameliorating a host of chronic diseases. The balloon technique as an imaginative method is a way of conveying new regulatory impulses to the body-mind-spirit complex.

This simple visualization helps to dissolve a client's tension while unblocking; it is much more efficient than massage techniques alone. It is especially suitable for painful conditions, movement restrictions, and functional disturbances. Using it enriches treatments and complements problem-solving in other contexts as well, because in all cases it enables new health strategies on the unconscious level.

Start by determining the point that needs to be unblocked. Then, holding that spot in your awareness, synchronize your breathing with your client's. Ask her to visualize that in that spot she is blowing up a balloon. Ask her the color of the balloon. When the balloon is nice and big, ask her to release the balloon, letting it lift up and fly away. In using this visualization be aware that the balloon is your client's, not yours. Avoid making any comments about color or any other properties of the balloon.

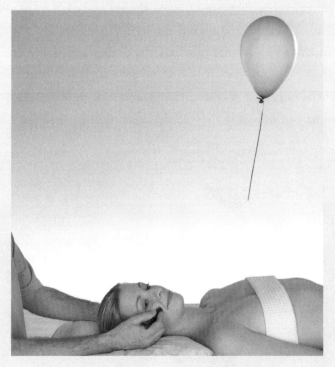

Basic unblocking with the balloon visualization, using a crystal wand

INCORPORATING ESSENTIAL OILS
IN REFLEXOLOGY

Essential oils take us into the realm of the emotions. We are delighted by the fragrance of a perfume, just as we are repelled by an ugly stench. This is due to the fact that our feelings are directly linked to our olfactory brain, which is important in deciding which foods are good for us and which ones are indigestible or even harmful. No matter where we apply them in reflexology massage, essential oils elicit our feelings, and since they are the finest essences of plants they influence all levels of being, body, mind, and spirit.

The many different essential oils have different properties. The oils of melissa, lavender, frankincense, Roman chamomile, and rose are calming, whereas the oils of rosemary, sandalwood, ginger, and bergamot bring more energy into the system. Oils also carry certain characteristics that we can regard as their "personalities." Since reflexology is a form of treatment that uses energy, the information encoded in the plant spirit of an oil is conducted through the reflexology zones to the organs. In this way essential oils have the ability to balance at all levels of a person's being.

Essential oils are very concentrated, and so if we were to apply them straight out of the bottle they could cause skin irritations. Therefore

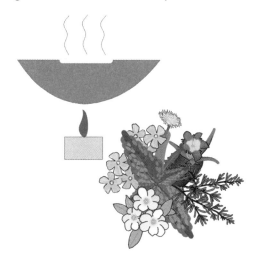

Essential oils balance
all levels of being.

it is best to dilute them with a neutral carrier oil in a ratio of 1:20 (1 part essential oil to 20 parts neutral oil). For larger area applications such as the back, a dilution of up to 1:50 is fine. Examples of suitable carrier oils are jojoba, almond, avocado, macadamia nut, and sesame. Use high-quality oils from a reputable source, since inferior oils can be contaminated and can harm or even reverse the desired healing effects of a treatment if they are not pure. Additionally, we must pay attention to possible allergic reactions and avoid any mucous contact. Therefore it is best to use kinesiology to test an oil on a client before using it.

In using essential oils in reflexology there are two options. One is to choose an oil for the entire treatment, a kind of theme. In this way we can influence the whole person. The second option is to select a specific oil for a disturbed zone. In each case we can find the right oil by muscle testing and checking for minimal clues. You can pour some neutral carrier oil in a hand and add one drop of the essential oil. Even better is to prepare an assortment of different essential oil dilutions in small bottles, an assortment of both calming and energizing oils. After calibrating for *yes* and *no,* hold a little bottle that contains an activating oil and then one with a calming oil directly on the zone and ask for a resistance of the thumb or the big toe. Alternatively, instead of contacting the zone we can touch the zone with one finger and wave the open bottle for one or two seconds under the nose of the client, then test, and then observe minimal clues. Then you'll know which oil is best for the overall treatment and which is best for the disturbed zones.

Next take three different oil dilutions of the appropriate energy direction, either activating or calming, and test for the best of the three. Apply a drop on the zone and massage it. Not much oil is needed in reflexology—less is best. The massage for diverting an abundance of energy is slow and gentle, whereas the one to enhance a decreased energy situation is faster and more vigorous. To remain below the pain threshold breathe to the rhythm of your client.

OVERVIEW OF ESSENTIAL OIL QUALITIES

Essential Oil	Mental/Emotional Properties	Physical Correspondences	Energy
Angelica	Strengthens our power reserves, increases courage, balances emotions	Autonomic nervous system, digestion, the heart and circulation	Strongly activating
Anise	Dissolves nightmares, eases feelings of loneliness and despair	Mucous membranes (particularly those related to digestion and breathing), menstruation	Calming
Bergamot	Raises spirits in cases of anxiety and diffidence	Digestion, urinary organs, the muscles	Slightly calming
Caraway	Calms hectic states of mind to help restore confidence	Digestion, mucous membranes, the muscles	Calming
Cardamom	Helps overcome depressive moods and reluctance	Digestion, circulation, hormonal regulation, the brain	Activating
Clary sage	Brightens sad/weepy moods, inspires creativity, quiets wearing thoughts, enhances sexual activities	Brain, lungs, skin, hormonal regulation; *contraindicated during pregnancy*	Slightly activating
Clover	Dissolves mental blockages and inner conflicts, reconciles oneself with unresolved experiences	Mouth (mucous membranes), teeth, digestion; *contraindicated during pregnancy*	Slightly calming
Cypress	Encourages clear decision-making, clears doubts, diffidence, and hesitancy	Lungs, muscles, joints, liver, gallbladder; *contraindicated during pregnancy*	Activating
Dill weed	Calms tempers and emotions, grounding	Digestion, the muscles (it was the oil of the Roman gladiators!), ears	Slightly calming
Frankincense	Concentrates one's soul forces, calms the mind and senses, quells overreactions	Muscles, heart, nervous system, digestion, breathing	Calming
Ginger	Encourages in times of fatigue, inspires and activates one's energies	Digestion, hormonal balance and sexuality, the joints and brain	Strongly activating

Essential Oil	Mental/Emotional Properties	Physical Correspondences	Energy
Lavender	Improves sleep, calms exceeding passions, helps with clear decision-making	Skin, ears, lungs, heart, and circulation	Calming
Marjoram	Relaxes in times of stress, soothes grief and despair	Mucous membranes, joints, digestion, lungs; *contraindicated during pregnancy*	Slightly calming
Melissa (lemon balm)	Calms nerves, fears, rage, and tempers; relaxes in times of stress; conveys peaceful serenity	Liver, gallbladder, heart and circulation, hormonal regulation	Calming
Mint	Supports mental regeneration and concentration, cheers mood	Brain, digestion, strong activator of the liver and gallbladder, hormonal regulation; *contraindicated during pregnancy*	Activating
Roman chamomile	Soothes all kinds of emotional tempests and nightmares, brings forth a comforting equanimity	Skin, muscles, heart and circulation, lungs, hormonal regulation	Strongly calming
Rose	Helps overcome lover's grief, opens the heart (especially after times of mourning)	Skin, blood, heart, hormonal regulation	Calming
Rosemary	Helps transfer thoughts into action and emotions into creativity	Skin, muscles, connective tissue, digestion, the heart and circulation	Strongly activating
Sandalwood	Supports overcoming fear and feelings of inferiority, enhances the appetite and laughing and happiness, helps release mental blockages	Skin, lungs, hormonal regulation (particularly male sex hormones); *contraindicated during pregnancy*	Strongly activating
Vetiver	Provides a foundation for thoughts and dreams, supports one's ideals, helps release depressive moods, increases sexual desire	Head, heart, skin, nervous system and senses, hormonal and sexual organs; *contraindicated during pregnancy*	Activating
Ylang ylang	Calms agitation, wrath, and disappointment; provides inner security and confidence; enhances harmony and sensuality	Head, heart, liver, skin, nervous system and senses, hormonal and sexual organs; *contraindicated during pregnancy*	Calming

CRYSTAL WANDS, THE PERFECT REFLEXOLOGY TOOLS

The shape of a crystal wand makes it perfectly suited and highly practical in reflexology treatments, and the healing properties of the different gemstones from which they are made provide an additional valuable dimension to the healing experience. I first discovered these amazing tools because I was looking for a way to go easy on my fingers in my massage work. The typical massage strokes in reflexology, especially those on the feet, can be a strain on the fingers, particularly on the joints of the thumbs. I have known many reflexologists who have had to quit their practice because of arthritis in these joints. I was also seeking more ways of making treatments energetically powerful. About twenty-five years ago I started experimenting with tumbled gemstones to explore their healing properties. I hit on the idea of carving massage tools out of these minerals and crystals. I had a few made, tried them, and loved the results, and from there crystal wands became integral to my practice. In the many years that I have been using them in reflexology treatments I have discovered a vast array of energetic properties of the different crystals and stones. Meanwhile these "tools of the trade" have become more widely accepted in other holistic modalities.

It is the shape and the minerals from which they are made that make crystal wands so special. They can be found in many variations but with one common feature: they taper from a strong, wide rounded end to a narrow rounded tip. This form makes them useful in reflexology, physiotherapy, acupressure, meridian massage, and chakra work. The thicker end can be used like a crystal sphere to support massage in large areas like the back or the soles of the feet, while the pointed end is suitable for working on minute reflexology points and on acupuncture points and trigger points.

Beyond their practical value to holistic practitioners are the possibilities offered by the energetic properties of the crystals themselves. In reflexology as in other holistic modalities there are two basic directions

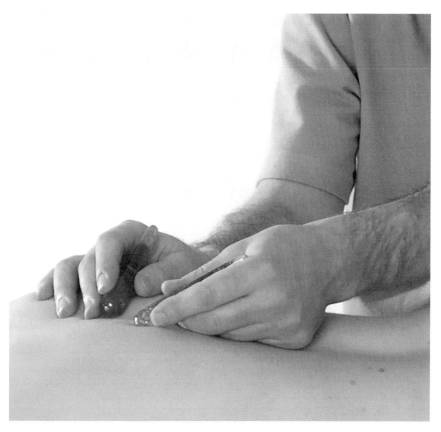

Reflexology gemstone treatments using two crystal wands

of energy needed to balance a disturbed reflexology zone and its associated organ: either activating to add energy to a depleted zone or calming
to diffuse a surplus of energy in an overactive zone. The lattice structure
of crystals endows them with specific qualities. For example, aventurine
has a diverting energy, as do amethyst, sodalite, and magnesite, to name
a few. On the activating side, to increase an energy level in a reflexology
zone there are, for example, red jasper, obsidian, bloodstone, and tiger
eye. The only truly neutral stone is rock crystal. This makes it the perfect
stone for use in the elevator technique, to search for disturbances.*

---

*For detailed information on how to work with crystal wands, see my book *Crystal
Wands: For Massage Therapy, Reflexology, and Energy Medicine.*

OVERVIEW OF CRYSTAL WAND QUALITIES

Gemstone	Mental/Emotional Properties	Physical Influences	Energy
Agate	Gives an enveloping feeling of security	Enhances elimination through the skin, stabilizes metabolism	Calming
Amazonite	Aids in coping with stress and bad tempers	Soothes tension and pain in muscles and joints	Calming
Amethyst	The crystal of peace, for calm alertness and profound consciousness	Alleviates headaches and nervous overreactions	Calming
Amethyst quartz	Clears the head and encourages sobriety, has a lifting effect on feelings of guilt and grief	Relieves pain	Calming
Apatite	Balances emotions: encourages in times of fatigue and calms excessive states	Benefits bones and teeth	Activating
Aquamarine	Balances discipline and stamina with ease and composure	*The* crystal for the eyes, balances hormones	Activating
Aragonite (brown)	A great mental stabilizer, lends flexibility in accomplishing tasks	Supports the liver, digestive system, and all structures of the spine	Slightly activating
Aventurine (green)	Encourages restful sleep by switching off thoughts, reduces nervousness	Soothes irritations of all kinds	Calming
Aventurine (red)	Promotes pragmatic drive, lends strength and internal security	Stimulates blood circulation, nerves, the senses, and sexual drive	Activating
Basalt	Like a stream of magma it slowly but surely develops our inner potential	Supports the entire metabolic process, promotes detoxification	Activating
Bloodstone (heliotrope)	Revitalizes in cases of exhaustion, alleviates irritability and impatience	Fortifies the immune system, relieves irritations and heart complaints	Activating

Gemstone	Mental/Emotional Properties	Physical Influences	Energy
Blue quartz	Calms the temper, helps with nervousness and stage fright	Reduces high blood pressure, alleviates pain	Calming
Bronzite	Conveys control and recovery in times of stress and challenge	Alleviates pain, dissolves tensions	Activating
Calcite (blue)	Supports efficiency in efforts required for a task	Eases issues with the lymphatic system, mucous membranes, skin, bones, and teeth	Calming
Calcite (orange)	Strengthens self-acceptance and self-confidence, lends a sunny inner warmth	Supports muscles, the gut and digestion, connective tissue, skin, joints, and bones	Activating
Carnelian	Opens the senses for humor and sociability	Activates blood circulation, stimulates the small intestine	Activating
Chalcedony (as blue-banded crystal)	Opens channels of communication, balances tempers, helps overcome inhibitions	Enhances the lymphatic system, the fluids of all glands, and kidney function	Slightly calming
Dolomite	Encourages new abilities, reduces stress, endows a sense of stability	Facilitates movement, alleviates tension and pain in muscles and joints	Activating
Dumortierite	"Take-it-easy" crystal, eases anxiety and depression	Reduces tensions, cramps, and headaches	Calming
Eldarite (kabamba)	Bestows inner strength, protects against negative influences	Strengthens the immune system, encourages regeneration, detoxifies (via perspiration)	Activating
Emerald	Intensifies alertness and clear vision for better understanding	Supports the liver and stimulates deacidification of the body	Activating
Epidote (unakite)	Helps overcome frustration and depression after failures	Supports regeneration and healing, strengthens the liver and kidneys	Activating
Feldspar (white)	Improves perception, attentiveness, and sensitivity	Enhances flexibility of tissues and muscles, regulates the female hormonal cycle	Slightly calming

Gemstone	Mental/Emotional Properties	Physical Influences	Energy
Fluorite	Increases flexibility, releases energetic blockages, enhances concentration	Beneficial for chronic issues with bones, joints, and mucous membranes	Slightly activating
Granite (all varieties)	Connects insights with experiences for successful realization of ideas	Stimulates digestion, metabolism, and circulation; alleviates back problems	Activating
Hematite	Lends willpower, vitality, endurance, and assertiveness	Supports formation of blood and transportation of oxygen within the body	Activating
Iron quartz	Sharpens the senses, allows adequate and swift responses to changes in the environment	Fortifies the autonomic nervous system, rejuvenates the skin	Activating
Jasper (red)	One of the strongest crystals of activity, dynamism, and courage	Stimulates circulation, activates all body functions	Activating
Labradorite	A healer crystal, supports intuition and mediumistic abilities	Cools conditions of excess, activates lethargic ones	Slightly calming
Lace agate	Lends flexibility and dynamic adaptability	Stimulates metabolism, digestion, and circulation	Slightly activating
Lapis lazuli	Brings self-confidence and self-awareness, fortifies a sense of responsibility, improves communication	Regulates hormonal glands, slows down the menstrual cycle	Activating
Larvikite (syenite)	Conveys a sense of calm sobriety and understanding helpful for problem-solving	Calms irritations, alleviates pain, encourages detoxification	Slightly calming
Lepidolite	Encourages focus on the essentials, brings inner peace, protects boundaries	Relieves pain associated with movement and the nervous system, soothes skin complaints	Calming
Magnesite	Improves patience, eases irritability and fearfulness	Relieves muscle cramps, headaches, and stomach complaints	Calming

Gemstone	Mental/Emotional Properties	Physical Influences	Energy
Magnetite	Strong activator, provides orientation in life and hones the ability to react	Activates energy in the body—especially in all glands, the liver, and the gallbladder	Activating
Mahogany obsidian	Lends power, initiative, and motivation; dissolves frustration and upsets caused by put-downs	Provides inner warmth, particularly for cold hands and feet; encourages wound healing	Activating
Malachite	Aids better and faster understanding of complex information	Relieves cramps, particularly in the sexual organs; and stimulates detoxification via the liver	Activating
Marble	Lends courage to change life circumstances and open oneself to new perspectives	Alleviates allergies; stimulates detoxification; strengthens the spleen, kidneys, and skin	Slightly calming
Mookaite	Encourages intense and happy experiences, balances the impulses	Cleanses the blood and strengthens the spleen, liver, and immune system	Activating
Moss agate	Relieves anxieties and feelings of depression, encourages hope and communication	Stimulates the immune system and lymph flow, detoxifies tissues	Slightly activating
Nephrite	Brings inner balance, alleviates impatience and grief, helps to make good decisions	Strengthens the kidneys, good for treating tinnitus and migraine	Slightly calming
Ocean jasper	Lends courage, encourages refreshing sleep, brings hope and confidence for the future	Good for lymph flow, the immune system, and regeneration after illness	Slightly activating
Onyx marble (aragonite calcite)	Calms and fortifies at the same time, conveys sensitivity for all rhythmic life processes	Eases spine problems and general joint complaints, supports the liver	Slightly calming
Petrified wood	Connects us to Earth, imparts a warm feeling of self-acceptance	Promotes digestion, detoxification, and elimination; good for losing excess weight	Activating

Gemstone	Mental/Emotional Properties	Physical Influences	Energy
Picasso marble (limestone)	Bestows solid grounding and objectivity, brings ideas into realization	Reduces water retention, supports the bones and intestinal activity	Slightly activating
Picture jasper (landscape)	Helps to persevere through situations of longstanding stress and to stand up again after failure	Supports digestion and elimination, cleanses the connective tissues, soothes allergies	Activating
Rhodonite	Healer crystal for body and soul, brings mutual understanding and friendship	Good for scars, connective tissues, and regeneration; encourages fertility	Activating
Rock crystal	The universally applicable neutral crystal for clarity, vitality, and awareness	Alleviates all kinds of pain, aids a more conscious perception of the physical body	Neutral
Rose quartz	Makes us sensitive, empathetic, and compassionate; encourages love and sexuality	Stabilizes the heart and blood circulation, helps with sexual and fertility difficulties	Slightly activating
Ruby in disthene (kyanite)	Boosts willpower and self-realization, mobilizes the spirit and life force	Good for nervous complaints, circulatory problems, and heart rhythm irregularities	Activating
Ruby in fuchsite	Promotes composure and responsibility, alleviates tensions, lends good sleep	Good for rheumatism, inflammation, and heart and back problems	Slightly activating
Sardonyx	Intensifies perception; lends friendliness, helpfulness, and inner balance	Strengthens the spleen and immune system, detoxifies, encourages lymph flow	Activating
Scolesite	Encourages team spirit, cools sexual urges, halts the draining of energy	Stabilizes the constitution, regenerates energy; good for the kidneys, bones, and ears	Slightly activating
Selenite	Shields against foreign influences, helps us retreat to find peace and rest	Dissolves hardness in muscles, soothes irritations and pain associated with movement	Slightly calming

Gemstone	Mental/Emotional Properties	Physical Influences	Energy
Septarian	Helps with staying steadfast in difficult situations while maintaining an open mind	Encourages deacidification and detoxification, dissolves hardening and growths	Slightly calming
Serpentine (all varieties)	Helps with mood swings, conveys a sense of protection, dissolves sexual blockages	Useful for heart rhythm irregularities and for kidney, stomach, and menstrual complaints	Calming
Smoky quartz	Classic antistress crystal to overcome burdens and internal tensions	Eases back problems and tight muscles, especially at the jaw	Calming
Snowflake obsidian	Dissolves states of shock, helps in overcoming lack of motivation and general fatigue	Increases blood circulation in the extremities, regenerates after accidents and operations	Activating
Snow quartz	Encourages attentiveness to your own potential, releases energetic blockages	Alleviates pain in the spine and all joints, supports the flow of all body fluids	Slightly calming
Sodalite	Creates free space and time for conscious changes and consistent self-development	Lowers fever and blood pressure, soothes irritations, supports water balance in the body	Calming
Stichtite in serpentine	Lends inner peace, balances turbulent emotions, conveys emotional openness	Strongly pain-relieving for rheumatic complaints, heart problems, and muscle cramps	Calming
Stromatolite	Helps adapt flexibility to new situations and grow with experiences	Improves digestion, metabolism, and intestinal flora	Calming
Sunstone	Promotes optimism, self-acceptance, and enjoyment of life; helps with anxieties and worries	Harmonizes the autonomic nervous system, stabilizes blood circulation	Activating
Tiger eye	Lends peace, composure, and courage to navigate through difficult times	Alleviates pain, calms the nerves, diminishes production of stress hormones	Activating

Gemstone	Mental/Emotional Properties	Physical Influences	Energy
Tiger iron	Mobilizes energy and provides new impulses for dynamic beginnings and developments	Stimulates blood formation and circulation, increases cellular vitality	Activating
Tourmaline, black (schorl)	Balances flow of energy in meridians, protects against energetic and psychic attacks	Alleviates pain and tensions, helps with numbness and the energetic unblocking of scars	Calming
Tree agate	Encourages inner peace, strength, and protection in times of challenge and change	Promotes vitality and a strong immune system, improves resistance to infection	Slightly activating

Using Crystal Wands

When using crystals wands in reflexology you will get the best results by selecting an appropriate crystal by way of muscle testing. Most likely you have already found the relevant reflexology zone to treat by testing in this way. Next test to see which direction of energy a point and its associated organ need. Is it activation or dispersion that brings the zone back into balance? To determine this simply hold an activating crystal on the point and ask for resistance of the thumb or big toe. Then switch to the other energy direction and hold a dispersing crystal on the point, repeating the request to resist. Remember, in using muscle testing it's just a slight resistance we seek, not a show of strength; the goal is to find out which direction of energy delivers the stronger hold. Once you have determined the direction take three crystals of the needed energy type and test to see which one is the best to use in the treatment.

For example, say we test the energy direction and determine the point and zone that need calming. Take an amethyst, a blue calcite, and an agate—three calming stones—and test again to see which is best for the treatment. The results of the muscle test will tell you which stone is needed.

Next use that stone in the basic unblocking procedure, slowly increasing the pressure on the zone until you get a change of breathing. At the moment you notice this signal stay with this amount of pressure on the point without moving the wand. After about ten to twenty seconds the person will visibly relax, breathe deeply, or even sigh. With this signal from the client lighten up on the point and gently stroke around in that zone with the crystal wand. This is done with the round end of the crystal wand.

With a lack of energy to the zone and associated organ the process is different. In this case you will activate the zone with the pointed end of the crystal wand, circling in a powerful but gentle mode. This should be comfortable and always without any pain.

5

......

Holistic Reflexology Treatments

TREATMENT CONSIDERATIONS

The abundance of reflexology systems highlighted in this book means that there is a treatment approach for almost any problem. For example, the feet are not attainable in foot reflexology, so we have to go to a different system for a twisted ankle. To soothe the ankle pain, reflexology on the ears on the feet zones would be the first choice (see page 35). Working on the feet zones on the skull would support the coordination of the muscle chains to relieve posture, and massage in the relevant dermatomes on the back would enhance communication from the nerve roots to the ankle.

We know that a twisted ankle does not occur without cause—there are components on the emotional and even the spiritual level. In the course of feeling angry about something perhaps the person might have stomped forward and not seen an obstacle on the ground; or maybe grief consumed him such that he didn't watch where he was going and tripped. Reflexology offers a gateway to the subconscious mind. Doing the balloon visualization in combination with massage of the foot

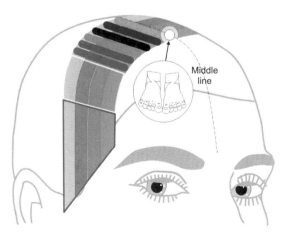

Reflexology treatments of the feet on the skull

points on the dermatomes of the back could open this man to understanding the unconscious motivations behind the trauma. The elegance in reflexology lies in networking between the various systems. Knowing more than just one system gives us a way to treat the body, mind, and spirit holistically. No matter whether it is an irregularity of the female hormonal cycle, back pain, headache, or just a professional massage to reduce tension, in all cases we can address the issue on different levels via two or three reflexology systems. The choice as to which systems to use is up to the practitioner, although muscle testing can be helpful in choosing which ones. Starting with the one that is most familiar we might find that after gaining some experience in that system we are attracted to other reflexology systems. They all follow the same basic approach to the flow of the energy.

There are, however, a few limitations to reflexology's ability to effectively address imbalances in the body; namely, in cases of extremely chronic, long-term illness. Nevertheless, even in such cases some soothing of pain or other improvements might be possible. The

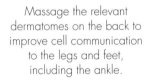

Massage the relevant dermatomes on the back to improve cell communication to the legs and feet, including the ankle.

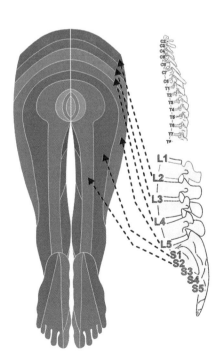

other obstacle to using reflexology effectively is when a person's tissues are completely blocked by a heavy accumulation of metabolic wastes, such that reflexology impulses do not resonate and treatment won't work. Metabolism refers to our inner primordial sea where our cells swim. At best our inner sea is as clear as the waters in an intact coral reef where we can see everything down to great depths. Here the nutrient carriers very easily find their delivery addresses, and our cells are

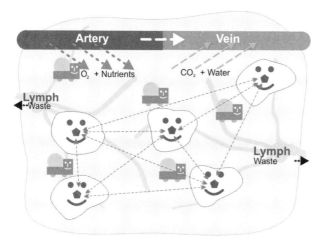

good metabolism

unhindered transfer of nutrients

efficient disposal of wastes

high-quality communication between the cells

A healthy metabolism lends itself to reflexology treatment.

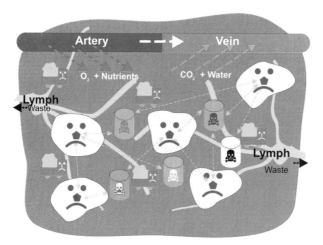

bad metabolism

restricted transport of nutrients

insufficient waste disposal

interrupted communication between the cells

In an unhealthy metabolism reflexology treatment will be relatively useless as the impulses will not resonate.

clearly recognized by the patrols of the immune system as members of our own body. The light signals of the cells reach their targets in a fast and error-free transmission.

Unfortunately our inner sea is often polluted. The metabolism can become overloaded due to many factors: pesticide residues in food and water, chemical colorings or flavorings in food, prescription medication residues—which the body cannot easily recover from—and the exhaust fumes of road traffic in urban areas. In such a loaded inner sea of metabolic wastes the integrity of the cells is compromised. The messengers no longer find all the delivery addresses, the cells are unhappy because they receive light signals from other cells in a distorted way, and the body's defense cells are suspicious because of all the unclear information; in their confusion they attack healthy cells or overreact to relatively insignificant substances. Examples are rheumatoid arthritis and allergies. At some point the body's compensatory reserves are exhausted, and functional losses develop from these chronic metabolic imbalances, which result in illness.

We all accumulate a certain amount of metabolic wastes as a consequence of modern life. Reflexology acts like a whisk in this kind of situation, whirling up the deposits, which are then removed via the kidneys, liver, and intestines. This is why it is important that reflexology treatments be accompanied by other complementary approaches to natural healing. On the day of treatment one needs to drink about one liter of additional water or tea that day than normal. Just by drinking enough water to flush the system of the whirled-up wastes, miracles can happen. In addition, one of the side effects of reflexology treatment is that all the excretory functions are activated: there is an increase in sweating, more intense urination, more frequent bowel movements, and the appearance of thin nasal mucus. These are all the short-term purification reactions of a healthy organism to the stimulation brought on by treatment and should be of no concern.

For those who take medication for conditions such as high blood pressure, heart problems, or diabetes, reflexology treatment can actually improve the bioavailability of those drugs. Because of this action diabetics are advised to check their blood-glucose levels more frequently than normal to avoid a drop in the blood-glucose level. And one should always seek medical attention if an ailment lasts longer than three days.

TREATMENT FOR HEADACHE

First the good news: about 90 percent of all headaches have harmless triggers. Nevertheless headaches are a nasty business, sometimes causing severe pain.

There are two types of headaches: primary headaches are not due to any recognizable cause, while secondary headaches occur due to another disorder, and the headache is simply a sign that something else is wrong in the body. It sounds contradictory, but taking painkillers can actually cause headaches, especially when there is a dull, helmetlike headache, in which case the choice of medication should be reconsidered. As well, other medications can cause headaches, especially blood-pressure medications. But the most common causes of headaches are fairly obvious: stress, dehydration, bad lighting, changes in the weather, sleep deficits, nocturnal teeth-gnashing, cigarette smoking (including secondhand smoke), alcohol, high levels of caffeine, and hormonal fluctuations within the female cycle are frequent triggers.

Migraine has multiple causes and is linked to spasms of the blood vessels in the brain induced by disorders of the autonomic nervous system. This causes edema around the vessels in the brain, resulting in tension in the head and neck, the source of pain. The neck muscles are very sensitive, and when irritated they interfere with the ultrasensitive autonomic-sympathetic nervous-system crosslinks; that is, the vertebral arteries and the connections to the cerebral nerves.

Reflexology is an effective treatment for migraine just as it is for the common headache. In fact reflexology may be able to prevent some of the secondary systemic symptoms of migraine, including nausea, dizziness, light and sound sensitivity, and aura.

There are several reflexology systems that are effective for the treatment of headache, including migraine. The best is hand reflexology. Self-massaging of the hands and along the thumbs, which correspond to the shoulder muscles and the cervical spine, brings at least some relief almost immediately. (See page 141.)

Foot reflexology treatment in the shoulders and cervical spine zones is also quite effective. (See page 142.)

Another important zone for treating headache, often overlooked, is the outside of the forearm just below the elbow of both arms. Gentle massage in these cervical zones is quite helpful even in acute situations. As well, a very promising approach is the region just inside the elbow. There the reflexology zones of the brain can be found. Even though there is not an exact map of the brain available on the inside of the forearm, treatment

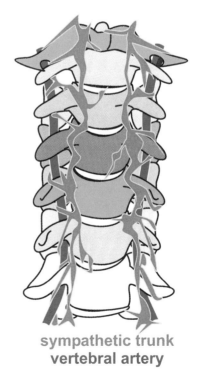

The sympathetic trunk and vertebral artery in the cervical spine

sympathetic trunk
vertebral artery

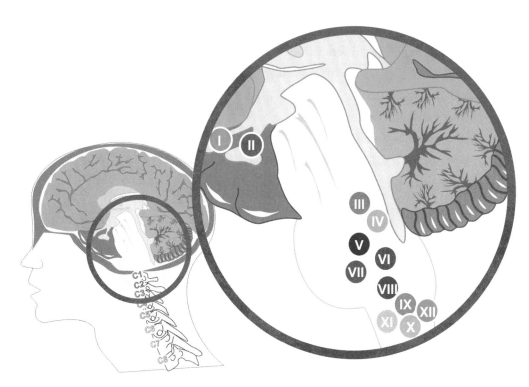

Olfactory nerve
for the sense of smell

Optic nerve
for the sense of sight

Oculomotor nerve
*for lifting the eyelid,
tension of the lens,
and eye movement*

Trochlear nerve
for eye movement

Trigeminal nerve
*for parts of the facial skin and parts of
the nose and the auricle,
lacrimal glands, ethmoid
teeth and tonsils, muscles of chewing,
tongue, floor of the mouth*

Abducens nerve
for eye movement

Facial nerve
*for tear glands, nasal mucosa, salivary glands,
taste buds, facial expression muscles;
also important for hearing*

Vestibulocochlear nerve
*for the sense of balance and
the refinement of the auditory sense*

Glossopharyngeal nerve
*for the parotid gland, swallowing reflex,
gustative sensations of the tongue,
connection to the circulatory and respiratory center*

Vagal nerve
*for regulation of the activity of most
internal organs, laryngeal and pharyngeal control,
transmitting of taste sensations*

Accessory nerve
*for the internal muscles of the larynx,
sternocleidomastoid muscle, and trapezial muscle*

Hyypoglossal nerve
for the function of the muscle of the tongue

Cerebral nerve nuclei in the brain stem and extended spinal cord there offers relief even in acute cases of migraine. (See page 143.)

One should always consider medical acupuncture, which can almost instantly bring relief from a headache when needles are applied to any of the points related to the cervical spine, the neck, and the shoulders, Meanwhile, if headache is a common occurrence, the first aim should be to find the triggers and change habits accordingly. Regular massage of the feet will bring overall relief of tension and break the vicious cycle of stress, tension, and head pain.

When using essential oils with reflexology for headache treatment we first have to take in to consideration the two possible states of energy— either a surplus or a lack of energy. If testing reveals a lack of energy

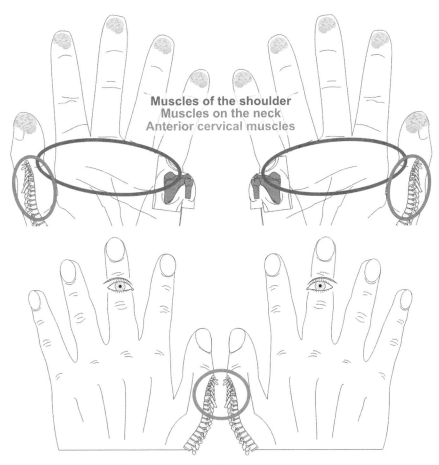

Reflexology treatments for head issues on the hands

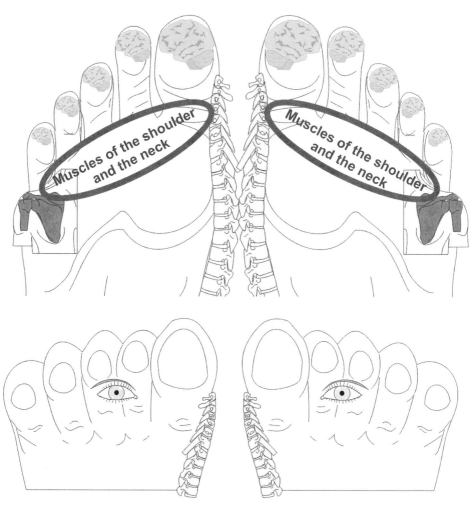

Reflexology treatments for head issues on the feet

we must activate with an essential oil such as ginger, mint, or cypress. These applications can be supported with crystal massages using lapis lazuli, rhodonite, ruby, or emerald. If testing indicates a surplus of energy associated with the headache we must calm the excessive energy state. Essential oils that can serve this purpose include melissa, frankincense, rose, and lavender. Amethyst, magnesite, aquamarine, or sodalite can be used for additional calming. When uncertain, a wand made of rock crystal is always right.

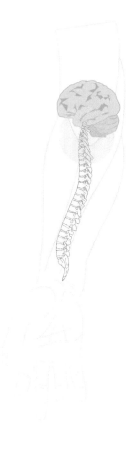

Reflexology treatments for head issues on the forearm and elbow

TREATMENT FOR SHOULDER AND JOINT PAIN

The shoulders are the most flexible joints of the body, with a great range of movement. That makes them prone to injury, wearing out, and distortion of the ligaments and muscles. The reason for a sudden pain in the shoulder in most cases is an overstretch or a tear of the joint capsule or tendon. Another cause of shoulder pain has its origin in the so-called impingement syndrome. This is the result of wear-related damage of the tendon of a muscle that passes through the narrowest part of the joint. All these syndromes don't need to result in inflammation of the tendons and other structures, but the symptoms—night pain, teeth-grinding, and restricted mobility—can be quite painful. One should note, however, that arthritis of the shoulder and the elbow is rather rare (whereas the hands, because of their extensive use, are subject to arthritis).

Foot reflexology treatment in the shoulder zones of both feet provides the fastest and easiest way to relieve shoulder pain.

The advantage of using foot reflexology as well as hand reflexology

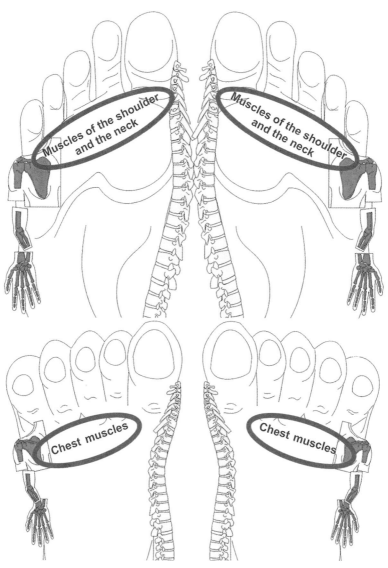

Reflexology treatment of the shoulder zones on the feet

to address shoulder issues is that we can precisely identify the zones of the shoulders on the feet and hands. Is the pain on the front of the shoulder? If so we can treat the upper side of the equilateral foot and hand. Pain on the back of the shoulder has its corresponding reflexology zone on the sole of the foot and the palm of the hand on the same side as the shoulder that is in pain. As an additional benefit massage of the feet in this zone helps boost the metabolism.

Not all problems with the upper limbs are in the body parts themselves. If that is the case we should try to find the real cause, particularly when physical therapy does not bring relief. In physiotherapy there is the phenomenon of referred pain, a felt pain in one area whose origin derives from a problem in another structure. Referred pain in the shoulders is a relatively common phenomenon. Due to a circuit fault in their switchover in the cervical spine, the signals give incorrect information about the true source of the pain. This is where consideration of the sclerotomes comes into play. Just by rubbing different spots on the bones we can determine which segment is involved. For example, we can differentiate the spinal influence by rubbing on the upper or lower side of the collarbone, since the upper side is supplied from segment C4 and the lower side gets its nerve impulses from C5 (see figure on page 146).

Shoulders, arms, hands—the upper limbs have the energetic function of reaching out, of protecting our personal space, and of literally handling the matters of our life. All of these are dependent on the flow of energy coming from our energetic center, the hara, just below the navel. In 1985, German diplomat, psychotherapist, and Zen master Karlfried Graf Dürckheim (1896–1988) made a convincing demonstration of this principle. For the demonstration, which took place on German television, Dürckheim asked for the participation of a young, healthy journalist. Dürckheim formed a ring with his thumb and index finger and then asked the journalist to pull them apart. That was easy for the young journalist. Then Dürckheim guided his chi force from his energy center into the ring of his fingers and asked the young man

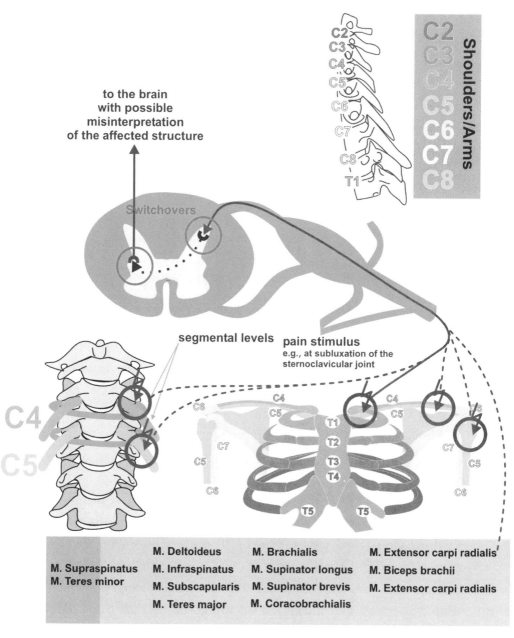

to the brain
with possible
misinterpretation
of the affected structure

Switchovers

Shoulders/Arms

C2
C3
C4
C5
C6
C7
C8

segmental levels   **pain stimulus**
e.g., at subluxation of the
sternoclavicular joint

M. Supraspinatus	M. Deltoideus	M. Brachialis	M. Extensor carpi radialis
M. Teres minor	M. Infraspinatus	M. Supinator longus	M. Biceps brachii
	M. Subscapularis	M. Supinator brevis	M. Extensor carpi radialis
	M. Teres major	M. Coracobrachialis	

Referred shoulder-pain phenomenon involves a fault in the switchover
in the cervical spine.

to try again to pull them apart. The look of astonishment on the journalist's face was quite obvious when he found that no matter how hard he tried, he could not pull the old man's fingers apart.

Another reflexology system that can address shoulder pain is found on the skull, where the hand zones have the biggest share of reflexology space. Elbows and shoulders are represented there as well, just a little smaller in comparison with the zones of the hands. But through testing we can find the relevant points for alleviating shoulder pain. Note that on the skull all reflexology zones are contralateral, meaning we find the zone for the right shoulder on the left side of the skull and vice versa.

Ear acupuncture by medical professionals offers yet another method of addressing shoulder issues (see page 148). One useful point that addresses all kinds of pain in general is the Shen Men, the "heavenly gate," one of the most recognized auricular points. This is the first point to be needled, followed by the point for the shoulder joint itself. In addition the ear's geometry according to Paul Nogier can be followed. This means drawing an imaginary line from the 0 point through

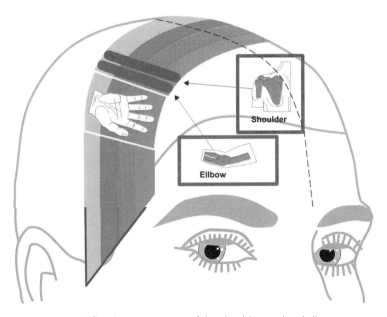

Reflexology treatments of the shoulder on the skull

the already pierced point to the outer rim of the ear. There we pierce another needle and go at an angle of 60 degrees to both sides once again to the rim of the ear. On each of the two points we also needle. Incidentally this procedure can be followed for other joint problems, including the hips, the knees, and the spine. If you do not use acupuncture it's worth treating these points on the ear with the tapered end of a crystal wand. French, Russian, and Chinese schools of ear acupuncture have differing opinions on whether the points on the ear should be treated on the same side as the problem or contralateral. The easiest solution is to treat both ears. If you want to be precise, test to determine the appropriate side for treatment.

For targeted treatments such as these it is necessary to determine which direction of energy a reflexology zone needs, whether activating or calming. This is particularly true when using essential oils and crystal

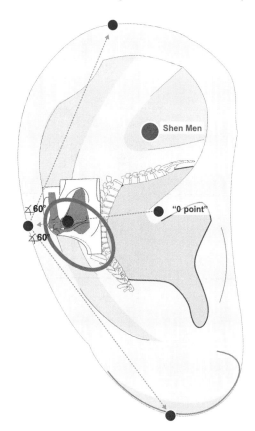

Auricular acupuncture points for shoulder pain

wands. Activating oils for the shoulder and upper limbs are rosemary and marjoram. Oils that diffuse excess energy are frankincense and dill (the latter was used by the Roman gladiators to relax their bodies after performing in the Colosseum). As for crystal wands, activating ones are fluorite and apatite, and to divert a surplus of energy use chalcedony and petrified wood. When in doubt work with neutral rock crystal.

TREATMENT FOR CARDIOVASCULAR HEALTH

Although the heart plays an important role in blood circulation its good functioning is not restricted to this organ alone. It is equally important to observe the condition of the arteries, the arterioles, and the capillaries. A slackening of their wall tension lowers the blood pressure, whereas their constriction results in a rise in blood pressure. Moreover, the entire regulation of our cardiac and circulatory system is highly dependent on the autonomic nervous system, which is closely connected to our feelings and to stress-related issues.

Our modern way of living is a huge burden on our cardiovascular system. The main culprit is stress. When it is a short-term alarm response it has no pathogenic effect. But ongoing stress can seriously harm the entire system, with consequences for body and spirit. The list of ailments resulting from stress is long and includes gastrointestinal problems, headache, tense muscles, depression, sleep disorders, immune deficiencies, sweating, heartburn, diabetes, chronic fatigue, heart palpitations, and cardiovascular disorders. Additionally the metabolism in the area of the capillaries, where the arteries turn in to veins, will be disturbed. This is where oxygen is released from the arteries for the cells, and carbon dioxide is taken over by the veins. Looking closer at stress we recognize a typical sequence of bodily functions. Knowing these makes it easier to understand how stress works and how to cope with it.

In a pre-phase of a stress response, when we see or hear something dangerous, the body abruptly winds down all metabolic processes. Most of the body's energies have to be made available for impending activation,

Parasympathetic nervous system with vagus nerve and abdominal nervous system

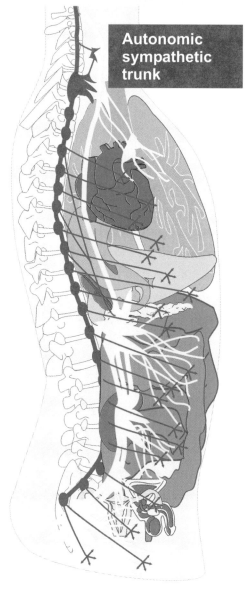

The parasympathetic nervous system

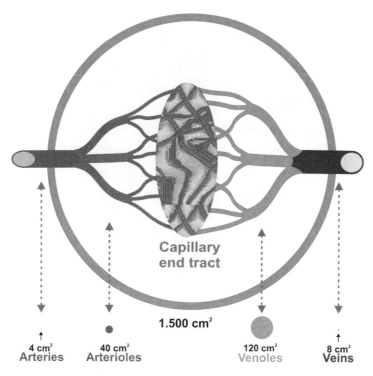

Proportional cross-sections in an arterial-venous supply area

for fight or flight. This response is sometimes perceived as fright associated with a halt in thinking and ineffectiveness in dealing with the demands of normal life. The next phase, alarm, is characterized by a release of the stress hormones adrenaline and norepinephrine. This phase mobilizes all energy with an acceleration of the heartbeat, tension of the muscles, changes in the blood chemistry, and a rise in blood pressure. Now the whole system is running in high gear. This response would be useful in times where quick action is needed, as when our ancestors had to escape from a saber-toothed tiger. Today the vicious cycle of stress is set into motion in any number of ways—a disturbing phone call, a driver who cuts us off, or discovering that we have no funds left in our checking account. When the stress response is activated there is no utilization of this energy by the muscles, as when escaping from the saber-tooth tiger. When this muscular response is missing the recovery phase of the stress reaction, with a normalization of the hormone level and replenishment of the reserves, is canceled as well. Then stress becomes a permanent inner state and can cause serious physical and mental problems. This chronic internal tension constricts the arterioles, and with an increase of resistance within the blood vessels the blood pressure rises.

Reflexology treatments have long-lasting effects on the autonomic nervous system; therefore they are excellently suited to support the regulation of the blood vessels. The systems that are particularly convenient for this purpose are the feet, the forearms, and the back. On the feet and on the forearms we treat the area of the brain stem. This is an important nerve center for regulating all our vital functions, including the autonomic nervous system. On the feet this zone is located exactly at the fold of the last joint of both big toes.

The technique for calming down a person by switching them over

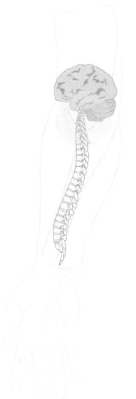

Reflexology treatment of the circulation on the forearm

from a stress mode to a relaxation mode is very easy. Just grab both big toes with a circle formed by thumb and index finger and hold the big toes pleasantly tight. Now execute a soft and cautious traction on the big toes and watch the respiration. At some point of pulling the breathing will change. Exactly at this moment hold this level of force and stay there. Eventually the person will take a deep breath or will sigh. This is the signal that the autonomic nervous system has switched over to relaxation mode. Afterward a nice general massage that includes the zones of the heart will further calm the person. The grip around the big toe is performed without essential oil, but you can apply a suitable oil for the overall massage of the feet.

The big-toe reach-around technique just described is also suitable for people who talk a lot, a sign of tension. With this technique the person will experience a decrease in tension and a quieter state of mind. The reflexology zones on the forearms for this nerve center are on the inside crook of the arm just below the elbow. It is always astonishing how fast people can unwind their stress level by gently

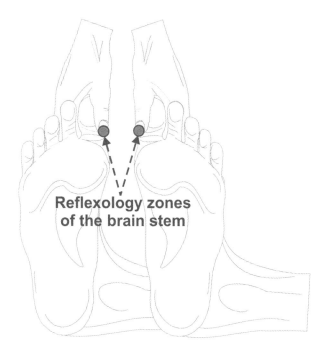

**Reflexology zones
of the brain stem**

Reflexology treatment
of the circulation on
the feet

massaging this area—a good thing to remember when there is a break in a conference or before an important business meeting. Adding a calming essential oil like lavender or rose is a nice addition to this kind of massage.

The heart is situated two-thirds on the left side and one-third on the right side in our chest. This location is mirrored on the back in the reflexology system there. With the exception of connective-tissue massage and acupuncture, which do require special training, learning how to do a nice reflexology massage of the back is relatively easy and doesn't require specialized training. Either with your finger or with the round end of a relaxing crystal wand stroke along the segments of the heart, beginning just beside the spine in the middle of the back as shown in the figure below. These gentle strokes are carried out along the space between the ribs all the way to the sides of the rib cage. Follow your intuition as to how many strokes in each area.

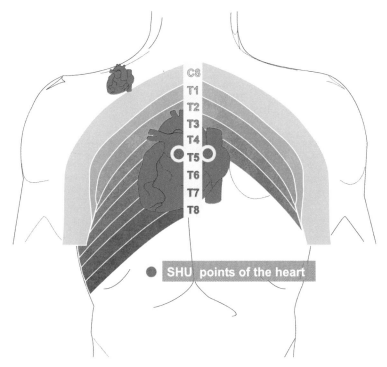

Reflexology treatment area for circulation on the back

If you use essential oils or crystal wands in the massage the aim is to calm energy, so the best oils are Roman chamomile, rose, lavender, and melissa; and the best stones are aventurine, malachite, rose quartz, and black tourmaline.

TREATMENT FOR DIGESTIVE HEALTH

There can be many reasons for being clogged-up, one of the most common digestive complaints. Lack of fiber in the diet and not enough exercise are only the most obvious causes of constipation, so first and foremost consider increasing physical activity and changing the diet. But to consider all the other factors involved in digestive problems let's take a closer look at this tube within us, which, at eight to ten meters in length, occupies a lot of space in the belly.

First of all, this tube always acts within the context of the whole organism, not in some isolated manner. Digestion starts in the mouth, where the food we eat becomes a chyme as a result of chewing and the action of saliva. This then moves to the other end of the tube, to the anal orifice, where wastes are discharged. What happens between these two points of entry and exit is what we call *digestion*. In the mouth is a kind of lab that analyzes food and sends its information to all parts along the tube: to the stomach, which furnishes acid and gastric enzymes; to the gallbladder, which prepares its juice, bile, to emulsify fat; to the pancreas, which provides its juice to crack carbohydrates, fats, and proteins and neutralize the acidity of the chyme moving through the system; to the small intestine, which organizes the assimilation of nutrients out of the chyme; and to the colon, which excretes wastes. Within this system all the different digestive organs are in close communication. Other organs and systems provide additional support to the digestive system: the liver, spleen, and the immune system, to name a few.

The immune system's task is not a minor one when it comes to digestion. GALT, gut-associated lymphoid tissue, mediates the immune

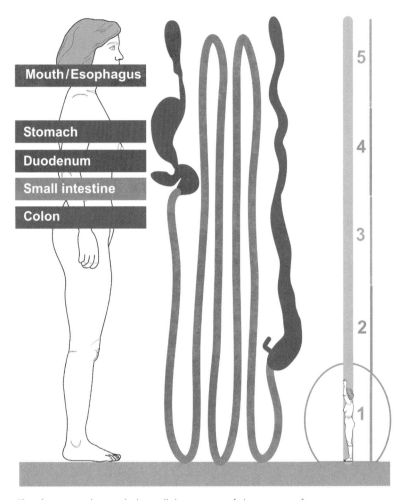

The digestive tube, including all the organs of digestion, is five times
as long as we are high with our arms stretched overhead.

response. For this reason any treatment of an infection, joint pain, and
food allergies and intolerances must address the digestive circuit. The
intestines contain about 100 trillion bacteria, double the number of
cells in the human body. We only know part of the story about how
these bacteria function and work together as it has only been relatively recently that microbiologists have had the tools that allow for
the investigation of our bacterial population and its interactions. The
colon in particular works as a fast breeder for bacteria: an examination

of stools shows that their composition is one-third bacteria, one-third cells that have scaled off from the inner walls of the intestines, and only one-third the remainders of food.

An interesting player in the digestive process is the enteric nervous system, called the "second brain"—one of the main divisions of the autonomic nervous system that consists of a meshlike system of neurons that governs the function of the gastrointestinal tract. This intestinal brain is capable of acting independently of the sympathetic and parasympathetic nervous systems, although it may be influenced by them. It consists of some 500 million neurons that are interwoven into all structures of the bowels. It encompasses all seven major chakras, or nerve centers, which are closely connected to the autonomic nervous system and are thus very susceptible to stress.

All these interrelationships have implications for the physical, mental, and spiritual levels of the organism. Any disturbance in one part of this complex system has implications for the entire body. This is why single-aimed measures taken to address stomach disorders, bile problems, constipation, or any other digestive difficulty mostly fail. For example, let's consider someone who has had their gallbladder removed because of gallstones. Bile is responsible for emulsifying fat in the chyme when it arrives in the duodenum, and bile acids accelerate the movement of the bowels. Normally when you eat something oily or a fatty piece of meat the analysis lab in the mouth communicates with the liver to produce more bile, which is stored in the gallbladder for later use. However, since this reservoir, the gallbladder, is gone, the bile flows directly into the duodenum. As a result the colon speeds up, and the person experiences frequent diarrhea after a meal because there is not enough bile juice available for good digestion. Other symptoms, besides frequent pooping, might include chronic fatigue, immune weakness, or symptoms like allergies, which we might never directly connect to the digestive system's trying to compensate for the absence of the gallbladder.

The complexity of digestion is an invitation for reflexology treatment, since regulation is its aim and its greatest strength. The best systems to use are the feet, the front of the torso, and the lower legs. For the feet it is beneficial to have a series of ten treatments a week. The feet are thoroughly massaged as a whole, with special strokes on the most conspicuous points. Oftentimes after the first two or three

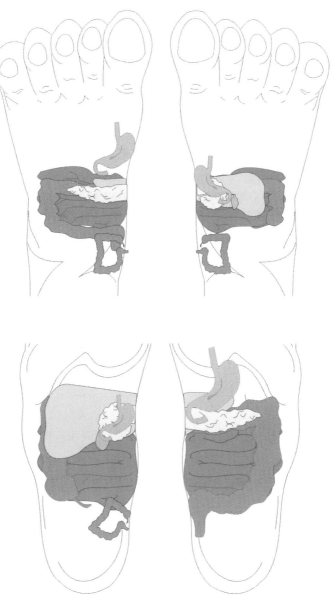

Foot reflexology treatment for digestion

treatments the person might experience slight diarrhea on the same day, but subsequently we can expect increasing normalization of the digestion, which has a positive influence on the overall health of the person.

Constipation and other uncomfortable sensations related to elimination are always connected to emotional blockages. The twelve reflexology points on the front of the torso corresponding to the Mu points

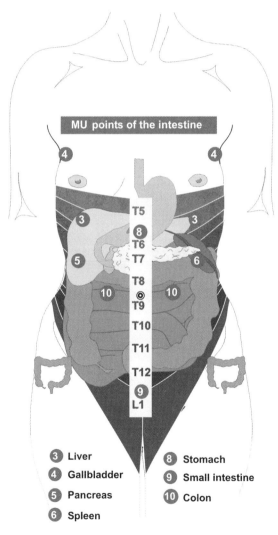

MU points of the intestine

T5
T6
T7
T8
T9
T10
T11
T12
L1

3 Liver
4 Gallbladder
5 Pancreas
6 Spleen
8 Stomach
9 Small intestine
10 Colon

Reflexology treatment of digestion on the front of the body

of traditional Chinese medicine are used to release congestion or tonify weak energy conditions in the digestive organs. The balloon visualization serves this purpose very well. Once the energies flow free again following reflexology treatment, the digestion makes itself audible with peristaltic bowel sounds. These sounds are always a good sign that there is a processing not only of the function of the intestines but also a release of the associated emotional and energetic blockages.

It's astonishing how fast the digestive system responds to just a little massage on the zones of the colon on the lower leg. Sometimes clients have to get up and run to the bathroom after just a few strokes. Here it should be pointed out that the effectiveness of treatment in

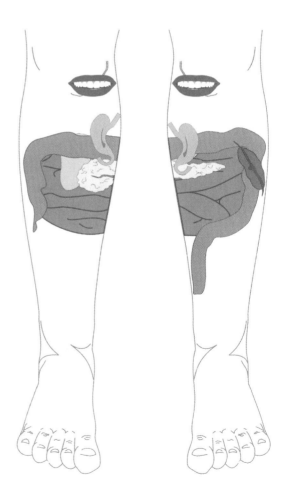

Reflexology treatment of the digestive system on the lower legs

these lower leg zones is not dependent on the amount of pressure applied; what is important is the connection to the energy center, the hara. When massaging here be very gentle with your hands.

In any treatment of the digestive system it is important to establish the direction of energy a zone needs, whether activating or calming, since we may have a blocked situation where energy needs to be supplied, or overactive bowels where we need to calm. This is an important consideration when it comes to using essential oils and crystal wands. Activating oils for the digestion are from marjoram, caraway seed, and clover; and calming oils are Roman chamomile and lavender. Activating crystal wands are picture jasper, red jasper, and orange calcite; and calming stones are dumortierite, smoky quartz, and serpentine.

Once equilibrium is restored to the digestive system it is important to consider how to maintain this balance. A balanced diet with a high proportion of fibers should be followed, and excessive sugar, salt, fast food, and carbonated drinks should be avoided, as all impair the digestion. Most people are not adequately hydrated, so proper hydration via water and herbal teas is crucial. Slow down when chewing food, and chew sufficiently. Physical activities like walking, hiking, and running work the iliopsoas muscles, providing an internal massage of the intestines.

TREATMENT FOR BACK PAIN

Apart from infection, back pain is the second most common reason why people go to see a doctor. Usually back pain is harmless and often disappears spontaneously after a few days of rest without any treatment. While some people suffer from back pain only occasionally, others experience it chronically.

There are many possible causes of chronic back pain, and the actual source of the pain cannot always be determined, even with x-rays and MRIs. Back pain can have an emotional component as well, and this is

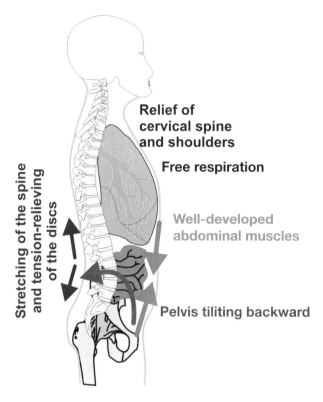

Good posture, including stability, is the key to maintaining the lumbar region in a state of health, as is good breathing.

not easily detected by technological means. In many cases, however, the cause of back pain is simply too little physical activity or weak muscles in the back and the abdomen, or a combination of both. Other factors are mental and even social issues, as surveys have shown that jobless people suffer more from lower-back pain than working people; as well, depression often goes hand-in-hand with back problems.

The spine has static and dynamic elements. The static elements are the vertebral and intervertebral discs. The dynamic elements are the ligaments, muscles, joint capsules, nerves, and the elaborate software that links all parts together to form a functional system. At every moment, lasting between twenty to seventy milliseconds, this software readjusts our posture to keep us upright on two legs, with the head in the uppermost position. We can compensate easily for minor disturbances in this play of forces, but chronic misalignment of the spine results in pain. The autonomic nervous system regulates the feedback loop that regulates equilibrium whether we bend forward, stand on one leg, or lie on the sofa. These functions are all connected to the sacroiliac joints and the hips. The interplay of these movement elements is also responsible for how basic energy is transferred around the body. This is what allows us to maintain a stable balance in life.

All of us have a little touch of scoliosis, which simply means that the spine is not ramrod straight but rather bent slightly to the one or the other side. This has to do with different muscle tension on either side of the body, where on one side the muscles are more tense and on the other side they are a little bit overstretched to compensate. In everyday life this is no problem, though we might notice the difference if we try to lift a box of water bottles up to a high shelf where we have to rotate the body. Under normal circumstances this might not pose a problem, but let's assume that we've just mowed the lawn on a sunny day with a light breeze, and we sweated with the exertion. The sweating in combination with the wind cooled down the muscles very rapidly, causing a functional disorder because of the sudden coldness. This causes us internal stress without our even realizing it. Now we try to lift that heavy box. The probability is high that we'll drop the box as we try to lift it, and for the next five to eight days we experience lower-back pain. This starts the vicious cycle of back tension, pain, more tension, and more pain. Even worse are the mental and emotional effects as we gradually lose a sense of balance in life.

Reflexology treatment addresses multiple aspects of this vicious cycle. It reprograms the body's software and brings the dynamic of the whole spine back into a balance. The systems that help best are the feet, the ears, and the iliac crest. A German medical masseur, Walter Froneberg (1932–2017), famously was able to readjust slipped discs by means of foot reflexology alone. He looked for the tensions in the

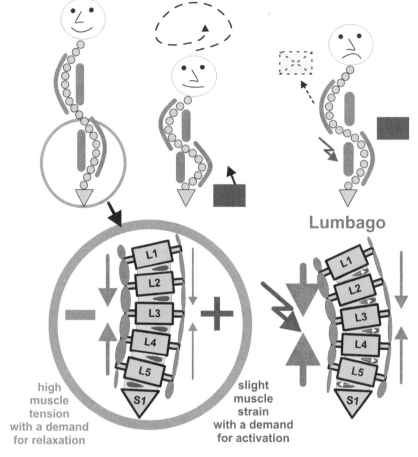

A little scoliosis is no problem under normal circumstances
but can cause pain when the back undergoes excessive strain.

different sections of the spine and activated or diminished the energetic situation according to the situation. The reflexology points referring to the tensed side of a vertebral section need a relaxing application, while the other side of the spine, the stretched side, needs activation. Such a procedure when performed on the zones of the feet balances the muscles of the spine and helps us maintain a permeability for the energies in our main pillar for upright posture. In the course of balancing the spine in this way, pain is soothed.

Auriculotherapy is another system that addresses lower-back pain.

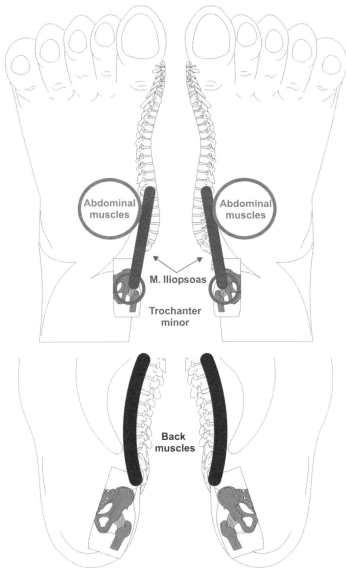

Foot reflexology treatment of the lumbar area

Neurologist Paul Nogier pioneered ear acupuncture out of curiosity. Nogier had a number of patients who had burn scars on the same spot on the ear. Upon inquiring he found out that they practiced an old method of the Gypsies, who would press the smoldering end of a twig

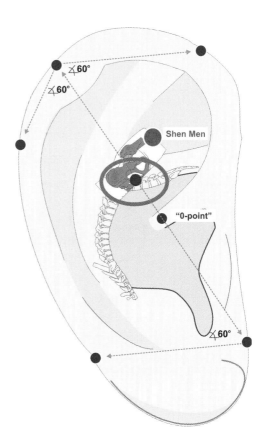

Reflexology treatment of the lumbar area by means of auriculotherapy

to that point to ward off back pain. We don't need to burn the ears anymore, because acupuncture of that spot or massaging with a crystal wand achieves the same effect. On the ears it is sometimes difficult to distinguish which side needs which energy direction. Test the relevant zones or points on both ears. This procedure is described in the shoulder section (pages 147–48).

The iliac crest is another good system to use for lower-back pain. At the iliac crest we can test the energy situation and work accordingly. At the end of the treatment use your knuckles and pull along the upper rim of the iliac crest from the front to the rear. It's best to put a few drops of an oil on that region before working deep with the knuckles. The best oils for the back are rosemary, sandalwood,

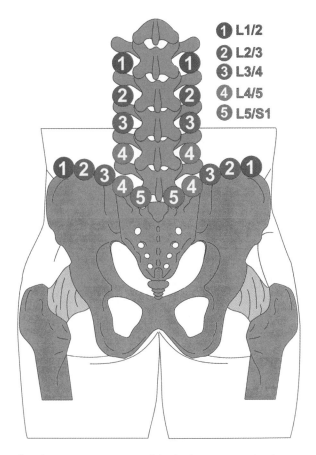

Reflexology treatment zones of the lumbar area on the iliac crest

and marjoram to activate, and frankincense or bergamot to divert energy away. Suitable activating crystal wands would be of obsidian or rhodonite, and for calming use petrified wood, black tourmaline, or magnesite.

All treatments for chronic back pain should be preceded by a thorough examination and followed by physiotherapy. Additionally it is always necessary to strengthen the abdominal muscles, to improve breathing, and to look in to possible mental and emotional components of the back pain.

CONCLUSION

From Practice to Healing Art

That all our knowledge begins with experience, there is no doubt.

IMMANUEL KANT

Experience has its root in doing and not in thinking alone. If there is no practical doing the knowledge that comes from experience will be missing. Then all thoughts will be dry ideas without any connection to the needs of life.

The aim of this book is in the direction of practice. By using all the possibilities that others have successfully proved through experience we gain knowledge from our common human heritage. This collective knowledge has long been present in our depths as a seed; we just didn't know it. This is about the awakening of healing abilities that are already dormant within us.

Whether we can develop a healing art from this practice depends on additional factors. For the ancient Greeks healing consisted of drawing conclusions from the observation of the visible signs of a disease and meeting the demands of the invisible factors. For us it is the same. Only in this way can we offer treatments that can soothe pain or cure a disease. This is the premise of the holistic approach that takes in to account all parts of the human being—physical, mental, emotional, and spiritual. These insights into the nature of illness and health also give us an opportunity to heal ourselves. Thus in this way our practice becomes a healing art.

I wish you much joy in exploring your abilities and in carrying health into your environment.

Bibliography

Adler, Ernesto. *Allgemein-Erkrankungen durch Störfelder: (Trigeminusbereich); Diagnose und Therapie.* Heidelberg, Germany: Verlag für Medizin Fischer, 1983.

Birdwhistell, Ray L. *Kinesics and Context: Essays on Body Motion Communication.* Philadelphia: University of Pennsylvania Press, 1970.

———. "The Language of the Body." In Silverstein, *Human Communication: Theoretical Explorations,* 203–20.

Bischof, Marco. "Biophotons: The Light in Our Cells." *Journal of Optometric Phototherapy,* March 2005, 1–5. www.biofieldimaging.com/uploads/1 /1/0/0/11003629/biophotons-the_light_in_our_cells.pdf.

David, Matthias. "Wilhelm Fliess (1858–1928): Die nasogenitale Reflextheorie." *Deutsches Ärzteblatt,* April 2007, 160–62. www .aerzteblatt.de/archiv/55192/Wilhelm-Fliess-(1858–1928)-Die -nasogenitale-Reflextheorie.

Dicke, Elizabeth. *Meine Bindegewebsmassage.* Stuttgart, Germany: Hippokrates -Verlag Marquardt, 1953.

Faure-Alderson, Martine. *Total Reflexology: The Reflex Points for Physical, Emotional, and Psychological Healing.* Rochester, Vt.: Healing Arts Press, 2008.

Feely, Richard A. *Yamamoto New Scalp Acupuncture: Principles and Practice.* Stuttgart, Germany: Thieme, 2010.

Fitzgerald, William H., Edwin F. Bowers, and George Starr White. *Zone Therapy.* Moke-lumne Hill, Calif.: Health Research, 1972.

Froneberg, Walter, and Gerda Fabian. *Manuelle Neurotherapie: Nervenreflextherapie am Fuss.* Heidelberg, Germany: Haug, 1992.

Garber, Miriam. *Iridology in Practice: Revealing the Secrets of the Eye.* Laguna Beach, Calif.: Basic Health Publications, 2013.

Gleditsch, Jochen M. *Mikro-Aku-Punkt-Systeme. Grundlagen und Praxis der somatotopischen Therapie.* Stuttgart, Germany: Georg Thieme, 2002.

Greenberg, Steven A. "The History of Dermatome Mapping." *Archives of Neurology* 60, no. 1 (2003): 126–31. doi:10.1001/archneur.60.1.126.

Haffelder, Günter. *Was unser Gehirn krank macht—Was unser Gehirn heilt.* DVD. Steinhardt, 2009.

Hecker, Hans-Ulrich., Angelika Steveling, and Elmar T. Peuker. *Microsystems Acupuncture: The Complete Guide; Ear-Scalp-Mouth-Hand.* Stuttgart, Germany: Thieme, 2006.

Horowitz, Sala. "Evidence-Based Reflexology: A Pathway to Health." *Alternative and Complementary Therapies* 10, no. 4 (2004): 211–16.

Hughes, Ciara M., S. Smyth, and Andrea S. Lowe-Strong. "Reflexology for the Treatment of Pain in People with Multiple Sclerosis: A Double-Blind Randomised Sham-Controlled Clinical Trial." *Multiple Sclerosis* 15, no. 11 (2009): 1329–38.

Ingham, Eunice D., and Dwight Byers. *Stories the Feet Can Tell Thru Reflexology and Stories the Feet Have Told Thru Reflexology.* 2nd ed. St. Petersburg, Fla.: Ingham Publishing, 1992.

Johnson, Elizabeth O., Themis C. Kamilaris, George P. Chrousos, and Philip W. Gold. "Mechanisms of Stress: A Dynamic Overview of Hormonal and Behavioral Homeostasis." *Neuroscience and Biobehavioral Reviews* 16, no. 2 (1992): 115–30.

Kliegel, Ewald. *Crystal Wands: For Massage Therapy, Reflexology, and Energy Medicine.* Rochester, Vt.: Healing Arts Press, 2018.

Kunz, Barbara, and Kevin Kunz. "Reflexology Paths Around the World." www.reflexology-research.com/?page_id=204/#hong-kong.

Leonhardt, Horst. *Fundamentals of Electroacupuncture According to Voll.* Translated by Helga Sarkisyanz. Uelzen, Germany: Medizinisch Literarische Verlagsgesellschaft, 1980.

Mandel, Peter, Judith Harrison, and Christopher Baker. *Acu-Impulsor Therapy: Treatment with Piezoelectric Impulses.* Portland, Oreg.: Medicina Biologica, 1988.

McDermott, R. "Profile: Ray L. Birdwhistell." *The Kinesics Report 2,* no. 3 (1980): 1–16.

McEwen, Bruce S., Nicole P. Bowles, Jason D. Gray, et al. "Mechanisms of Stress in the Brain." *Nature Neuroscience* 18, no. 10 (2015): 1353–63. doi: 10.1038/nn.4086.

Müller, Wolf, Günter Haffelder, Angelika Schlotmann, et al. "Amelioration of Psychiatric Symptoms through Exposure to Music Individually Adapted to Brain Rhythm Disorders: A Randomised Clinical Trial on the Basis of Fundamental Research." *Cognitive Neuropsychiatry* 19, no. 5 (2014): 399–413.

Nóbrega, Carlos A. M. da. "Biophoton: The Language of the Cells. What Can Living Systems Tell Us about Interaction?" *Technoetic Arts: A Journal of Speculative Research* 4, no. 3 (2006): 193–202.

Newsweek. "The Biology of Beauty." June 2, 1996. www.newsweek.com/biology -beauty-178836.

Nogier, Paul. *De l'auriculothérapie à l'auriculomédecine.* Paris: Maisonneuve & Larose, 1999.

Park, Jae W. *A Guide to Su Jok Therapy.* Lancaster, UK: Gazelle Distribution Trade, 2003.

Petty, Nicola J. *Principles of Neuromusculoskeletal Treatment and Management: A Guide for Therapists.* Edinburgh: Elsevier Churchill Livingstone, 2004.

Pischinger, Alfred. *Das System der Grundregulation: Grundlagen für eine ganzheitsbiologische Theorie der Medizin.* Heidelberg: Haug, 2009.

Pischinger, Alfred. *The Extracellular Matrix and Ground Regulation: Basis for a Holistic Biological Medicine; Basics for a Holistic Biological Medicine.* Edited by Hartmut Heine. Translated by Ingeborg Eibl. Berkeley, Calif.: North Atlantic Books, 2007.

Sanches, Andrea, Rafaela Costa, Fernanda Klein-Marcondes, and Tatiana Sousa-Cunha. "Relationship among Stress, Depression, Cardiovascular and Metabolic Changes and Physical Exercise." *Fisioterapia em Movimento* 29, no. 1 (2016): 23–36.

Schiffter, Roland, and Elke Harms. *Connective Tissue Massage: Bindegewebsmassage According to Dicke.* Stuttgart, Germany: Thieme, 2014.

Schlegel, Emil. *Die Augendiagnose des Dr. Ignaz von Péczely.* N.p.: CreateSpace Independent Publishing Platform, 2015.

Seaman, David R., and Carl Cleveland III. "Spinal Pain Syndromes: Nociceptive, Neuropathic, and Psychologic Mechanisms." *Journal of Manipulative Physiological Therapeutics* 22, no. 7 (1999): 458–72.

Sharkey, John. *The Concise Book of Neuromuscular Therapy: A Trigger Point Manual.* Chichester, U.K.: Lotus Publishing, 2008.

Siener-Stiftung, Rudolf, and Christian Schütte. *NPSO: Erfolg mit der Neuen Punktuellen Schmerz- und Organtherapie.* Oberfranken, Germany: Mediengruppe, 2011.

Silverstein, Albert, ed. *Human Communication: Theoretical Explorations.* London: Routledge, 2015.

Strobl, Anton. *Die Zungendiagnostik als Hilfsmittel des praktischen Arztes.* [*Nach einem Vortrag auf der 12. Tagung der "Arbeitsgemeinschaft für Erfahrungsheilkunde" in Bad Brückenau am 4. Mai 1957*]. Heidelberg, Germany: Haug, 1974.

Tae, Woo Yoo. *KHT Koryo Hand Therapy: Korean Hand Acupuncture.* Vol. 1. Seoul, Korea: Eum Yang Mek Jin, 2001.

Tiran, Denise. *Clinical Reflexology: A Guide for Integrated Practice.* London: Elsevier Churchill Livingstone, 2010.

Voeikov, Vladimir L., R. Asfaramov, E. V. Bouravleva, et al. "Biophoton Research in Blood Reveals Its Holistic Properties." *Indian Journal of Experimental Biology* 41, no. 5 (2003): 473–82.

Voll, Reinhard. *Topographische Lage der Messpunkte der Elektroakupunktur.* Uelzen, Germany: Medizinisch Literarische Verlagsgesellschaft MBH, 1976.

Yamamoto, Toshikatsu, and Thomas Schockert. *Yamamoto New Scalp Acupuncture.* Bad Koetzting, Germany: Verlag Systemische Medizin, 2005.

Zeitler, Hans. *Einführung in die Schädelakupunktur.* Heidelberg, Germany: Haug, 1977.

Zeitler, Hans, and Johannes Bischko. *Handbuch der Akupunktur und Aurikulotherapie / Einführung in die Schädelakupunktur.* Heidelberg, Germany: Haug, 1978.

Zhang, Yingqing. *ECIWO Biology and Medicine: A New Theory of Conquering Cancer and a Completely New Acupuncture Therapy.* Huehaote Neimenggu, China: Neimenggu People's Press, 1987.

Zong Xiao-fan, and Gary Liscum. *Chinese Medical Palmistry: Your Health in Your Hand.* Boulder, Colo.: Blue Poppy Press, 1995.

Index

Page numbers in *italics* indicate illustrations.